Oxford Specialist Handbooks in
Cardiology

Heart Failure

Roy S. Gardner
Scottish National Advanced Heart Failure Service,
Glasgow Royal Infirmary,
Glasgow, UK

Theresa A. McDonagh
Royal Brompton and Harefield NHS Trust,
London, UK

Nicola L. Walker
Department of Medical Cardiology,
Western Infirmary,
Glasgow, UK

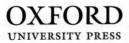

OXFORD
UNIVERSITY PRESS

OXFORD

UNIVERSITY PRESS

Great Clarendon Street, Oxford OX2 6DP

Oxford University Press is a department of the University of Oxford.
It furthers the University's objective of excellence in research, scholarship,
and education by publishing worldwide in

Oxford New York

Auckland Cape Town Dar es Salaam Hong Kong Karachi
Kuala Lumpur Madrid Melbourne Mexico City Nairobi
New Delhi Shanghai Taipei Toronto

With offices in

Argentina Austria Brazil Chile Czech Republic France Greece
Guatemala Hungary Italy Japan Poland Portugal Singapore
South Korea Switzerland Thailand Turkey Ukraine Vietnam

Oxford is a registered trade mark of Oxford University Press
in the UK and in certain other countries

Published in the United States
by Oxford University Press Inc., New York

British Library Cataloguing in Publication Data

Data available

Library of Congress Cataloging in Publication Data

Data available

Typeset by Newgen Imaging Systems (P) Ltd., Chennai, India
Printed in Italy
on acid-free paper by
LegoPrint S.p.A.

ISBN 978-0-19-920573-8 (flexicover: alk.paper)

10 9 8 7 6 5 4 3 2 1

Oxford University Press makes no representation, express or implied, that the drug
dosages in this book are correct. Readers must therefore always check the product
information and clinical procedures with the most up-to-date published product
information and data sheets provided by the manufacturers and the most recent
codes of conduct and safety regulations. The authors and the publishers do not
accept responsibility or legal liability for any errors in the text or for the misuse or
misapplication of material in this work. Except where otherwise stated, drug dosages
and recommendations are for the non-pregnant adult who is not breast-feeding.

Foreword

The '39' steps of heart failure

Running to no fewer than that number of chapters, this book, like its eponymous forebear is intriguing, eminently readable and, ultimately, very satisfying. It is an 'A to Z' of the condition which is now the commonest cardiovascular cause for emergency admission to hospital. Far from accusing contemporary medicine of failing people with heart failure, this stark statistic simply states that heart failure is the price that an ever increasing number of people pay for the success of modern cardiovascular medicine. Thus, heart failure is the direct result of better detection and treatment of its most common underlying causes, formerly hypertension and valve disease, and more recently, coronary heart disease. Together with the societal changes in modern democracies these 'medical' factors combine to allow more of us to grow old enough to expose our hearts and blood vessels to the consequences of the ageing process.

Published in 2007, this book is timely for it is in this very year that heart failure has gained official recognition within the wider cardiovascular community by being listed as one of the 5 subjects for sub-specialty training in cardiology alongside percutaneous coronary intervention, electrophysiology, adult congenital heart disease, and imaging. There could be no better handbook to serve as a road map for all trainees in their new training programmes than this new offering in the highly successful Oxford Specialist Handbooks in Cardiology. But it will not just be young cardiologists who will benefit from this highly informative resource because its concise readable style will prove attractive to the broad spectrum of healthcare professionals who care for people with heart failure especially general, care of the elderly and primary care physicians, specialist heart failure nurses, pharmacists, rehabilitation and palliative care specialists.

Heart failure is, in every sense, a 'big' subject. It affects millions of people worldwide, has many diverse causes, is informed by a large number of 'megatrials' of several classes of medicines and devices, is extremely costly due to the huge number of hospital bed days it uses, is complicated by many co-morbid conditions, and occupies an untold number of healthcare professionals in its management.

Unsurprisingly therefore any attempt at comprehensive coverage of such a vast canvas, necessarily, needs a grand vision. *Heart failure* succeeds in its scope, scale, clarity, and its sheer informativeness. From the standpoint of the healthcare professional in the various theatres of practice this excellent publication will not only educate them thoroughly about heart failure, it will also guide them in the practical aspects of actually how to perform the diagnostic tests, do the procedures, calculate the infusion rates or doses of medications, and look after the patient properly.

This book also reminds us constantly that heart failure is not simply a diagnosis suggested by symptoms and confirmed by an echocardiogram but is the clinical reflection of the detrimental effects on the heart and circulation of almost any disease of the heart. Too often this simple fact is forgotten in the rush to manage patients by protocol rather than taking the time to treat each patient as an individual who deserves an accurate diagnosis in order to develop an appropriate management plan. Evident throughout this book is the need for a multidisciplinary approach in order to decide whether to advise palliation, carefully titrate complex medication to target doses, or initiate complex investigations when the prospect of a potentially remediable cause seems credible.

Dr Theresa McDonagh and her duo of Specialist Registrars have produced what is possibly the most concise but comprehensive account of both acute and chronic heart failure that has been published to date. It will be widely read and constantly referred to by all those who care for people with heart failure.

Professor Henry Dargie
Consultant Cardiologist and Director of the
Scottish National Advanced Heart Failure Service

Preface

Heart failure is an important and ever expanding sub-speciality of cardiology. Many health care professionals are now developing specialist expertise in heart failure. This is true for cardiologists in training, consultant cardiologists, care of the elderly and general physicians, cardiothoracic surgeons, primary care doctors, pharmacists, and specialist nurses.

With advances in medical therapy, the prognosis of the condition has improved dramatically. Whereas once heart failure was a pre-terminal diagnosis, now for many it is treatable. However, some patients remain symptomatic and at high risk of death despite maximal medical therapy. These patients can now benefit from a range of novel devices and other advanced therapies.

Heart failure is an extremely complex condition to both diagnose and manage. This is due in particular to the large burden of co-morbidities involved. This has made multi-professional delivery of heart failure care essential to achieve the best outcomes for patients.

This book aims to cover comprehensively all aspects necessary to manage a patient with heart failure. It gives simple, clear advice on the diagnosis, investigation, and treatment options available. The book is set out logically to mirror the patient journey in heart failure.

The chapters provide concise and objective information to guide all health care professionals involved in the modern day multi-disciplinary management of the syndrome. In addition it is also designed to be an effective training manual for cardiology juniors and trainees in heart failure specialist nursing programmes. As such, we hope that this book, in the easy to use Oxford Handbook style, will serve as the flagship manual of heart failure management that addresses the needs of all the health care team.

Our ultimate desire is that it facilitates the practice of optimal evidence-based management of heart failure to improve outcomes for our patients.

RSG
TAMcD
NLW
June 2007

Acknowledgements

Firstly, we would like to acknowledge those closest to us for their patience whilst we were writing this book. Allan McPhaden kindly provided the histopathology images. We would also like to acknowledge the following people for their role in proof reading chapters of our book: Roger Carter, Clare Gardner, Laura Laing, David McCarey, David McGrane, Andrew Murday, and Robyn Smith.

RSG
TAMcD
NLW
June 2007

Contents

Section VI How to set up and run a heart failure service

Section VII End of life issues

Symbols and abbreviations

⚠	warning
►	important
►►	don't dawdle
🖋	controversial topic
♂	male
♀	female
↑	increase
↓	decrease
→	leading to
📖	cross reference
ACC	American College of Cardiology
ACE	angiotensin converting enzyme
ACEi	angiotensin converting enzyme inhibitor
ACTH	adrenocorticotrophic hormone
ADP	adenosine diphosphate
AF	atrial fibrillation
AHA	American Heart Association
A-HeFT	African-American heart failure trial
AHF	acute heart failure
AHI	apnoea–hypopnoea index
AIRE	acute infarction ramipril efficacy study
ANP	atrial natriuretic peptide
Ao	aorta
AR	aortic regurgitation
ARB	angiotensin receptor antagonist
ARVC	arrhythmogenic right ventricular cardiomyopathy
AS	aortic stenosis
AT_1	angiotensin II type-1
ATG	antithymocyte globulin
ATII	angiotensin II
ATLAS	assessment of treatment with lisinopril and survival
AV	atrioventricular
AVNRT	atrioventricular nodal re-entry tachycardia
AVRT	atrioventricular re-entry tachycardia
BiPAP	bi-level positive airway pressure support
BiVAD	biventricular assist device

BK	bradykinin
BMD	Becker muscular dystrophy
BP	blood pressure
CABG	coronary artery bypass grafting
CHARM	candesartan in heart failure: assessment of reduction in mortality and morbidity
CHB	complete heart block
CHD	coronary heart disease
CHF	chronic heart failure
CIBIS	cardiac insufficiency bisoprolol study
CMR	cardiac magnetic resonance
CNS	central nervous system
CO	cardiac output
COMET	carvedilol or metoprolol European trial
COMT	catechol-O-methyl transerase
CONSENSUS	cooperative North Scandinavian enalapril survival study
COPERNICUS	carvedilol prospective randomized cumulative survival study
COX	cyclo-oxygenase
CPAP	continuous positive airways pressure
CPET	cardiopulmonary exercise testing
CRT	cardiac resynchronization therapy
CRT-D	cardiac resynchronization therapy-defibrillator
CRT-P	cardiac resynchronization therapy-pacing
CSA	central sleep apnoea
CT	computer tomography
CTR	cardiothoracic ratio
CTx	cardiac transplantation
CVP	central venous pressure
DAD	delayed after depolarization
DAVID	dual chamber and VVI implantable defibrillator
DIG	Digitalis Investigation Group
DMD	Duchenne muscular dystrophy
DNA	deoxyribo nucleic acid
EAD	early after depolarization
ECG	electrocardiogram
ECMO	extracorporeal membrane oxygenation
ecNOS	endothelial cell NOS
EDTA	ethylene diamine tetraacetic acid
EEG	electroencephalogram
ELITE	evaluation of losartan in the elderly study

EMF	endomyocardial fibrosis
EMG	electromyography
EPHESUS	eplerenone post–acute myocardial infarction heart failure efficacy and survival study
ESC	European Society of Cardiology
FDA	Food and Drug Administration
FEV_1	forced expiratory volume in 1 second
FVC	forced vital capacity
Gd	gadolinium
GFR	glomerular filtration rate
HCM	hypertrophic cardiomyopathy
HCP	health care professional
HDL	high-density lipoprotein
HES	hypereosinophilic syndrome
HF	heart failure
HIV	human immunodeficiency virus
HLA	human leukocyte antigen
IABP	intra-aortic balloon pump
ICD	implantable cardiac defibrillator
IL	interleukin
ISDN	isosorbide dinitrate
IVD	interventricular delay
IVS	interventricular septum
LA	left atrial
LBBB	left bundle branch block
LDL	low-density lipoprotein
LIDO	levosimendan infusion versus dobutamine
LV	left ventricular
LVAD	left-ventricular assist device
LVEDP	left ventricular end-diastolic pressure
LVEF	left-ventricular ejection fraction
LVNC	left ventricular non-compaction
LVOT	left ventricular outflow tract
LVSD	left-ventricular systolic dysfunction
MAO	monoamine oxidase
MAOIs	monoamine oxidase inhibitors
MDRD	modification of diet in renal disease
MERIT-HF	metoprolol CR/XL randomized interventional trial in heart failure
MMF	mycophenolate mofetil
MR	mitral regurgitation

MS	mitral stenosis
MTWA	microvolt T-wave alternans
NIPPV	non-invasive positive pressure ventilation
NSAID	non-steroidal anti-inflammatory drug
NYHA	New York Heart Association
OSA	obstructive sleep apnoea
PA	pulmonary artery
PAC	pulmonary artery catheter
PCWP	pulmonary capillary wedge pressure
PDEI	phosphodiesterase inhibitor
PLVEF	preserved LV function
PMBV	percutaneous mitral balloon valvotomy
PND	paroxysmal nocturnal dyspnoea
PPCM	peripartum cardiomyopathy
PR	pulmonary regurgitation
PS	pulmonary stenosis
PVR	pulmonary vascular resistance
PVRI	PVR index
RA	right atrium
RhA	rheumatoid arthritis
RAAS	renin–angiotensin–aldosterone system
RALES	randomized aldactone evaluation study
REMATCH	randomized evaluation of mechanical assistance for the treatment of congestive heart failure
RER	respiratory exchange ratio
REVIVE	randomized multi-centre evaluation of intravenous levosimendan efficacy
RNVG	radionuclide ventriculography
RV	right-ventricular
RVAD	right ventricular assist device
SAM	systolic anterior motion
SAVE	survival and ventricular enlargement study
SAVER	surgical anterior ventricular endocardial restoration
SCA	senile cardiac amyloidosis
SCD	sudden cardiac death
SDC	serum digoxin concentrations
SENIORS	study of the effects of nebivolol intervention on outcomes and re-hospitalization in seniors with heart failure
SHFM	Seattle heart failure model
SLE	systemic lupus erythematosis

SNP	sodium nitroprusside
SNS	sympathetic nervous system
SOLVD	studies of left ventricular dysfunction
SPECT	single photon emission computed tomography
SPWMD	septal-to-posterior wall motion delay
SUPPORT	study to understand prognoses and preferences for outcomes and risks of treatments
TAH	total artificial heart
TDI	tissue Doppler imaging
TM	thrombomodulin
TNF-α	tumour necrosis factor-α
TPG	trans-pulmonary gradient
TPMT	thiopurine methyltransferase
TR	tricuspid regurgitation
TRACE	trandolapril cardiac evaluation study
TS	tricuspid stenosis
TV	tricuspid valve
UF	ultrafiltration
VAD	ventricular assist device
Val-HeFT	valsartan-heart failure trial
Vd	volume of distribution
V_E	minute ventilation
VMAC	vasodilation in the management of acute CHF
V_T	ventilatory threshold

Section I

Chronic heart failure

Definition, epidemiology, and pathophysiology

Definition

Physiological—inability of the heart to pump sufficient oxygenated blood to the metabolizing tissues despite an adequate filling pressure.

Working clinical definition—clinical syndrome consisting of symptoms such as breathlessness, fatigue, and swelling of ankle caused by cardiac dysfunction.

Chronic heart failure (CHF) can be caused by any type of cardiac dysfunction and is most commonly attributable to left-ventricular dysfunction. Only rarely does a patient present with CHF as a result of isolated right-ventricular (RV) dysfunction. RV dysfunction is usually secondary to LV dysfunction and its sequelae.

The most common and best-studied cause of CHF is left ventricular systolic dysfunction (LVSD), although CHF also occurs in the presence of preserved systolic function. Left ventricular systolic dysfunction is relatively easy to diagnose by a range of non-invasive methods. The diagnosis of CHF with preserved left ventricular ejection fraction (LVEF) is more difficult (☐ Chapter 20). It is often attributed to diastolic dysfunction, although abnormalities of systolic and diastolic function frequently co-exist. To prove diastolic dysfunction, invasive haemodynamics are necessary, but many non-invasive tests can infer its presence.

Classification

Heart failure (HF) can present either as a chronic condition or acutely, occurring *de novo* or as a decompensation of chronic heart failure. Acute HF is covered in ☐ Chapters 23 and 24.

Current US guidelines also classify patients into the following stages:

Stage A Those at high risk of developing HF, for example, hypertensives, diabetics.

Stage B Patients with structural cardiac disease or remodelling who have not yet developed HF, that is, asymptomatic LV dysfunction.

Stage C Patients with current or prior HF symptoms.

Stage D Those with end-stage HF.

This system emphasizes the need for prevention of the development of heart failure in the first place due to aggressive risk factor control. It also highlights the importance of treating asymptomatic LVSD to prevent its progression to symptomatic LVSD, that is, CHF.

Key references

McDonagh TA et al. Symptomatic and asymptomatic left-ventricular systolic dysfunction in an urban population. Lancet 1997; **350**: 829–33.

McKee PA et al. The natural history of congestive heart failure: the Framingham study. N Engl J Med 1971; **285**: 1441–6.

Erikson H et al. Risk factors for heart failure in the general population: the study of the men born in 1913. Eur Heart J 1989; **10**: 647–56.

Redfield MM et al. Burden of systolic and diastolic ventricular dysfunction in the community: appreciating the scope of the heart failure epidemic. JAMA 2003; **289**: 194–202.

Hunt SA et al. ACC/AHA 2005 guideline update for the diagnosis and management of chronic heart failure in the adult: a report of the American college of cardiology/American heart association task force on practice guidelines (writing committee to update the 2001 guidelines for the evaluation and management of heart failure). J Am Coll Cardiol 2005; **46**: e1–82.

Epidemiology

Prevalence

- Using clinical criteria, CHF prevalence 1–2% of population.
- ♂ > ♀.
- Increased in the elderly (approximately 15%).
- European population-based studies of LVSD show:
  - Prevalence of 2–3%.
  - Increasing to 7% in the elderly.
- Approximately ~50% of patients with significant left ventricular systolic dysfunction have no symptoms or signs of heart failure (**asymptomatic LVSD**).
- Prevalence of HF with preserved LVEF 9.7/1000 (44% of the total HF prevalence).
- Range of prevalence for HF with preserved LVEF varies from 15 to 50%.

Incidence

- The Framingham heart study (USA) results state that annual incidence of 0.2–0.3% in those aged 50–59 years, increasing 10-fold in those aged 80–89 (Fig. 1.1).
- The UK population data is similar, with an annual incidence of 0.12% in those aged 55–64, rising to 1.2% in those aged over 85. Median age of presentation is 76 years.
- ♂ > ♀, particularly due to LVSD.
- HF with preserved LVEF occurs more among:
  - Elderly individuals
  - Women
  - African Americans.

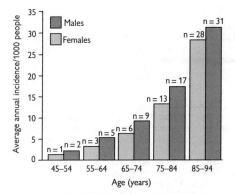

Fig. 1.1 Incidence of heart failure. Reproduced from McKee PA *et al.* The natural history of congestive heart failure: the Framingham study. *N Engl J Med* 1971; **285**: 1441–6 with permission from Massacheussets Medical Society.

Aetiology

- There is geographical variation.
- In Westernized societies, two-thirds are secondary to ischaemic heart disease.
- Other important contributors are:
  - Hypertension
  - Valve disease
  - Alcohol.
- Rheumatic disease is the most common cause in the developing world.
- Chagas disease is an important cause in South America (📖 Chapter 19).
- Hypertension is an important factor in Africans and African Americans. It is proportionally more common in heart failure with preserved LVEF.
- There has been a shift in the aetiology over time in long-term population-based studies such as Framingham.
  - Decreased importance of hypertension.
  - Increased relevance of ischaemic heart disease (Fig. 1.2).

Causes of chronic heart failure

- Coronary heart disease
- Hypertension
- Valve disease
- Congenital heart disease
- Infective: for example, viral myocarditis, Chagas, HIV, Lyme disease
- Alcohol
- Toxins: for example, anthracyclines, abstruzimab
- Deficiencies: for example, selenium, beri beri, thiamine
- Haemochromatosis
- Idiopathic
- Familial
- Peripartum
- Tachycardia induced
- Infiltrative states: amyloid, sarcoid, endomyocardial fibrosis, hypereosinophilic syndrome
- High output: for example, A–V fistulae, Paget's disease

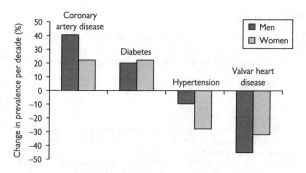

Fig. 1.2 The changing pattern of aetiology of CHF in the Framingham study with time. Reproduced from McMurray JJ & Stewart S. Epidemiology, aetiology, and prognosis of heart failure. *Heart* 2000; **83**: 596–602 with permission from BMJ Publishing Group Ltd.

Prognosis

The prognosis in CHF is poor. Population-based studies report significantly lower survival rates than those seen in heart failure treatment trials.

- The mortality from CHF at 5 years in the Framingham study (32-year follow up).
  - 62% in men
  - 42% in women.
- UK data (Fig. 1.3):
  - Six-month mortality rate 30%
  - Over 40% do not survive 18 months from the time of diagnosis.
- Mortality rates are in excess of many common solid malignant tumours (breast, prostate, colon, and melanoma).
- Population-based studies: survival of HF with preserved LVEF is better.
- Hospitalized patients with HF with preserved LVEF: similar mortality rates to those patients with LVSD.
- CHF is extremely disabling, with frequent and recurrent hospitalizations.
- CHF reduces quality of life to a greater extent than other chronic medical disorders including arthritis and stroke.
- CHF is an expensive condition, consuming 1–2% of total NHS expenditure in the UK.

Trends in epidemiology

CHF is projected to increase in prevalence by 50% in the next 20 years. The prevalence and incidence of CHF are rising due to:

- Changing demography of the population, that is, more elderly at risk.
- Improved survival of other cardiovascular diseases, for example, MI.
- Improved survival rates for CHF.

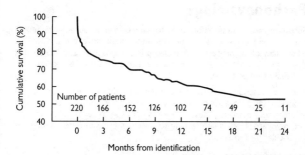

Fig. 1.3 Mortality after a first diagnosis of heart failure. Reproduced from Cowie MR et al. Survival of patients with a new diagnosis of heart failure: a population based study. *Heart* 2000; **83**: 505–10 with permission from BMJ Publishing Group Ltd.

Key references

Ho KK et al. The epidemiology of heart failure: the Framingham study. *J Am Coll Cardiol* 1993; **22**: 6A–13A.

Cowie MR et al. Survival of patients with a new diagnosis of heart failure: a population based study. *Heart* 2000; **83**: 505–10.

Levy D et al. Long-term trends in the incidence of and survival with heart failure. *N Engl J Med* 2002; **347**: 1397–402.

Pathophysiology

Sustained cardiac dysfunction leads to haemodynamic, autonomic, neuro-humoral, and immunological abnormalities. These drive the pathway to CHF. Many of the processes are maladaptive, originally designed to protect the organism from exsanguination and hence to maintain blood pressure and vital organ perfusion.

The best-described mechanisms are the activation of various neurohor-monal systems. In addition, there is intense activation of cytokines and inflammatory markers. These processes combine to cause fluid retention and myocardial cell death leading to a vicious cycle of deteriorating left ventricular performance.

Haemodynamics

Decreased cardiac output leads to the following:
- ↑ Left ventricular end-diastolic pressure (LVEDP).
- ↑ Pulmonary capillary wedge pressure (PCWP).
- The development of pulmonary oedema.

PCWP is a poor correlate of symptoms because other factors also contribute.

Initially, increased filling pressures augment ventricular performance early in the disease process (Frank Starling law), but as the increased filling pressures persist, the myocardium fails and cardiac output drops.

The renin–angiotensin–aldosterone system (RAAS)

Decreased cardiac output decreases renal afferent arteriolar blood flow, causing secretion of renin and production of angiotensinogen and angiotensin I. This is converted in the lung by the angiotensin converting enzyme (ACE) to the octapeptide, angiotensin II (ATII) (Fig. 1.4).

ATII is a major effector hormone of this system, causing the following:
- Vasoconstriction
- Myocyte hypertrophy and fibrosis
- Aldosterone release
- Activation of noradrenaline and endothelin.

Aldosterone causes sodium- and water-retention and hypokalaemia resulting in the following:
- Pulmonary and peripheral oedema
- Myocardial cell loss via apoptosis
- Myocardial fibrosis
- Increased afterload.

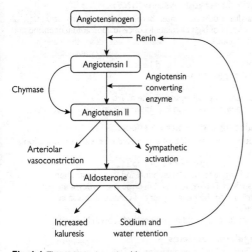

Fig. 1.4 The renin–angiotensin–aldosterone system.

Key reference

Swedberg K. Importance of neuroendocrine activation in chronic heart failure. Impact on treatment strategies. *Eur J Heart Fail* 2000; **2**: 229–33.

The sympathetic nervous system (SNS)

Decreased cardiac output activates baroreceptors causing activation of the SNS. The effects of high circulating concentrations of epinephrine and norepinephrine include

- ↑ Heart rate.
- ↑ Blood pressure.
- ↑ Myocardial oxygen demand.
- Toxic effects on the myocardium—cell death.
- Down-regulation of β_1 receptors in the heart.

There is a concomitant decrease in parasympathetic nervous activity.

Other circulating and paracrine effects

Other circulating and paracrine effects include increased production of the following:

- Endothelin: a potent vasoconstrictor peptide.
- Vasopressin: leading to water-retention and vasoconstriction.
- Cytokines such as TNF-α, IL-1, and IL-6 causing myocyte apoptosis which contribute to the development of cardiac cachexia in advanced HF.
- Increased circulating steroid hormones and growth hormone.

Counter-regulatory systems

Not all the hormonal systems activated in CHF are deleterious. Various counter-regulatory mechanisms to oppose sodium- and water- retention are also activated, for example, the natriuretic peptide system.

The natriuretic peptide system

Myocardial pathology and the increased wall stress caused by a raised LVEDP and LA pressure, lead to LV and LA wall stretch and the secretion of the natriuretic peptide hormones (Fig. 1.5). These natriuretic peptides cause

- Natriuresis.
- Vasodilatation.
- Offset the activation of the RAAS and SNS.

Two types of natriuretic peptide circulate in high concentrations in HF:

- Brain natriuretic peptides (Fig. 1.6)
  - BNP, the active peptide
  - NT-pro-BNP, the inactive N-terminal cleavage fragment.
- Atrial natriuretic peptide (ANP and NT-ANP).

Adrenomedullin, another natriuretic hormone is also produced and circulates in higher concentration. When heart failure progresses the more powerful negative effects of the RAAS and SNS outweigh these beneficial processes.

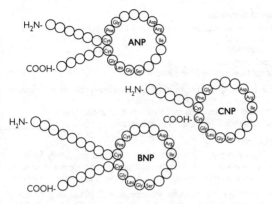

Fig. 1.5 The natriuretic peptides from *Heart Failure in Clinical Practice* (2nd edition) edited by McMurray J & Cleland J. Martin Dunitz Ltd, London, 2000, (Figure 5.1) with permission from Taylor and Francis.

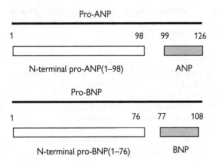

Fig. 1.6 Cleavage of pro-hormones of BNP and ANP into active peptides and inactive N-terminal fragments.

Key reference

Rademaker MT & Richards AM. Cardiac natriuretic peptides for cardiac health. *Clin Sci (Lond)* 2005; **108**: 23–36.

Peripheral changes

Abnormalities of skeletal muscle occur in CHF, including
- Wasting.
- Impaired perfusion.
- Increased fatigueability.
- Abnormal histology and metabolism.

These correlate with symptoms of fatigue, exercise-intolerance, and poor prognosis. These changes may be secondary to
- Physical inactivity, anorexia and poor intestinal absorption.
- Insulin resistance, TNF-α, and norepinephrine.

Arrhythmias

The CHF syndrome is associated with an increased propensity for both atrial and ventricular arrhythmias. In particular, the development of atrial fibrillation (AF) can contribute to the further deterioration of LV function.

There are multiple mechanisms for arrhythmias in CHF, including structural changes, ischaemia and neurohormonal activation (□ Chapter 11). Additional factors such hypo- and hyperkalaemia, hypo- and hypermagnesaemia, drug interactions, and toxicity may precipitate arrhythmias.

Co-morbidities

CHF is frequently associated with co-morbidities that can lead to progression and deterioration. These can occur due to the HF syndrome, the treatment, or due to other diseases, for example, diabetes.

The commonest co-morbidities are
- **Renal dysfunction**: eGFR <50mL/minute is present in 20–50% of all HF patients. It may be caused by reduced renal perfusion, the effects of drugs or co-morbid conditions such as renal artery stenosis, hypertension, and diabetes. The presence of renal dysfunction increases both morbidity and mortality in CHF (□ Chapter 17).
- **Anaemia**: This is present in up to 40% of those with advanced HF. It can be anaemia of chronic disease or due to iron deficiency often associated with aspirin and chronic GI blood-loss. Anaemia is also associated with increased morbidity and mortality in CHF (□ Chapter 13).

Intercurrent cardiac events

Progression of CHF can also be caused by further myocardial insults, for example, MI, ischaemia (causing hibernation and stunning), hypertension, valvular regurgitation or stenosis, or arrhythmia.

Progressive LV remodelling

These processes cause sodium- and water-retention, and depression of myocardial performance. This ultimately leads to adverse remodelling of the left ventricle: a process involving myocyte hypertrophy, death, and fibrosis.

In CHF with LVSD, this inexorable progression of the syndrome leads to a dilated, spherical ventricle. The natural history of this so-called 'cardiovascular continuum' (Fig. 1.7), starts early on with risk factors for heart disease, which leads to MI, and LVD, is the end stage of the syndrome—death occurs either from progressive pump failure or suddenly, often as a consequence of ventricular arrhythmia.

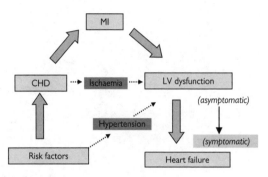

Fig. 1.7 The cardiovascular continuum.

Key references

Bristow MR. Why does the myocardium fail? Insights from basic science. *Lancet* 1998; **352**(Suppl I): SI8–14.

Weber KT. Aldosterone in congestive heart failure. *N Engl J Med* 2001; **348**: 1689–97.

Mann DL & Young JB. Basic mechanisms in congestive heart failure. Recognising the role of pro-inflammatory cytokines. *Chest* 1994; **105**: 897–904.

Wilson JR Mancini DM & Dunkman WB. Exertional fatigue due to skeletal muscle dysfunction in patients with heart failure. *Circulation* 1993; **87**: 470–5.

Chapter 2

Diagnosis and investigation

Introduction

Heart failure is a clinical syndrome: a constellation of symptoms and signs that are ultimately due to cardiac dysfunction.

▶ CHF is not a diagnosis, and a cause for the underlying cardiac dysfunction must always be sought and treated, if possible.

There are two aspects to the diagnosis and investigation of HF:
• Confirmation of the presence and type of cardiac dysfunction.
• Ascertainment of the cause of that cardiac dysfunction.

A thorough investigation to search for the co-morbidities that often accompany heart failure should be pursued. These are possible precipitants of decompensation, which may affect its subsequent management.

Diagnosis of HF

Clinical symptoms and signs

The cardinal symptoms and signs of HF are
- Breathlessness.
- Fatigue.
- Peripheral oedema.

Breathlessness is usually exertional, but in more advanced cases appears at rest. Orthopnoea and paroxysmal nocturnal dyspnoea (PND) may occur especially in the presence of pulmonary oedema.

Physical signs can be present and relate either to the presence of fluid retention and/or poor cardiac output. They can include
- Sinus tachycardia.
- Atrial fibrillation or other arrhythmia.
- Hypotension.
- Increased JVP.
- Ankle and sacral oedema.
- Pulmonary crackles.
- Signs of pleural effusion.
- Displaced apex beat.
- Hepatomegaly.
- Ascites.
- Third and/or fourth heart sounds.
- Murmurs.

The important point about these clinical symptoms and signs is that they raise the suspicion of heart failure. Clinical acumen alone leads to an inaccurate diagnosis of HF in up to 50% of cases. The symptoms and signs are either both over-sensitive and non-specific or, if they are specific, lack sensitivity. Symptoms are used to assign an NHYA class to patients (Tables 2.1 and 2.2).

▶ The presence of cardiac dysfunction must be proved to make the diagnosis.

Table 2.1 New York Heart Association (NYHA) classification of heart failure

Class I	No limitation; ordinary exercise does cause undue dyspnoea, fatigue, or palpitation
Class II	Slight limitation of physical activity; comfortable at rest but ordinary activity results in dyspnoea, fatigue, or palpitation
Class III	Marked limitation of physical activity: comfortable at rest but less than ordinary activity results in dyspnoea, fatigue, or palpitation
Class IV	Unable to carry out any physical activity without discomfort; symptoms of heart failure are present even at rest with increased discomfort with any physical activity

Table 2.2 Sensitivity and specificity of clinical symptoms and signs in heart failure

Clinical features	Sensitivity (%)	Specificity (%)
Breathlessness	66	52
Orthopnoea	21	81
PND	33	76
History of oedema	23	80
Tachycardia	7	99
Pulmonary crackles	13	91
Oedema on examination	10	93
Third heart sound	31	95
Raised JVP	10	97

Adapted from Sosin M *et al. A Colour Handbook of Heart Failure. Investigation, Diagnosis and Treatment.* Mansion Publishing, 2006, with permission from Blackwell.

Guidelines for the diagnosis of HF

Recognized guidelines (ESC, ACC/AHA, NICE, SIGN) all state that to diagnose HF the following should be present (Fig. 2.1):
- Symptoms and or signs of heart failure.
- Cardiac dysfunction at rest.
- Response to treatment if the diagnosis is in doubt.

Investigation of suspected heart failure

- **12-lead ECG**: HF is rare in the presence of a normal ECG. The negative predictive value of the ECG is >90%.
- **B-type natriuretic peptide** (BNP or NT-proBNP): a value within the normal range has an extremely high negative predictive value (>98%) for the exclusion of HF (see Fig. 2.4).
  - Increased values indicate either a cardiac functional/structural abnormality or renal dysfunction.
  - BNP/NT-pro-BNP concentrations:
    — ↑ with age in normals.
    — higher in ♂ than ♀.
    — age–sex corrected normal values may aid diagnosis.
  - Increased BNP/NT-pro-BNP concentrations need further investigation and cardiac assessment.
- **CXR**: A normal chest x-ray does not exclude a diagnosis of heart failure as the cardiothoracic ratio (CTR) is normal in 50% of cases.
  - Cardiomegaly (CTR >0.50) may be suggestive of a cardiac abnormality, particularly with evidence of pulmonary congestion.
  - Helps to identify and exclude other causes of breathlessness.

Diagnosis of cardiac dysfunction

LV function is usually assessed non-invasively by **echocardiography**. The types of cardiac dysfunction (i.e. myocardial, valvular, or pericardial) should be identified. Other modalities can be used, for example, nuclear techniques, cardiac MR or invasive contrast ventriculography at cardiac catheterization.

For myocardial dysfunction the detection of systolic dysfunction is a crucial preliminary step. The most common way of expressing myocardial performance is by the calculating the LVEF.

$$\text{LVEF (\%)} = \frac{\text{LV diastolic volume} - \text{LV systolic volume}}{\text{LV diastolic volume}} \times 100.$$

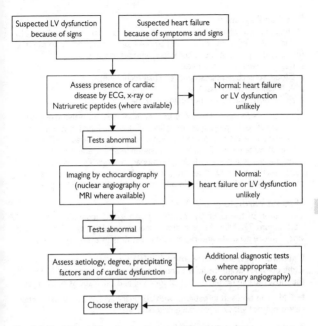

Fig. 2.1 The ESC guidelines for the diagnosis of HF and LV dysfunction. Reproduced from Swedberg K *et al.* Guidelines for the diagnosis and treatment of chronic heart failure: executive summary (update 2005): the Task Force for the Diagnosis and Treatment of Chronic Heart Failure of the European Society of Cardiology. *Eur Heart J* 2005; **26**: 1115–40 with permission from Oxford University Press.

Key references

Swedberg K *et al.* Guidelines for the diagnosis and treatment of chronic heart failure: executive summary (update 2005): the Task Force for the Diagnosis and Treatment of Chronic Heart Failure of the European Society of Cardiology. *Eur Heart J* 2005; **26**: 1115–40.

Hunt SA *et al.* ACC/AHA 2005 guideline update for the diagnosis and management of chronic heart failure in the adult: a report of the American college of cardiology/American heart association task force on practice guidelines (writing committee to update the 2001 guidelines for the evaluation and management of heart failure). *J Am Coll Cardiol* 2005; **46**: e1–82.

NICE Guideline for Heart Failure: www.nice.org.uk

Echocardiography

LV function and dimensions are usually determined by echocardiography. An accurate LVEF can be obtained by the biplane Simpson's rule method[*] (Fig. 2.2). Simpler and more common methods include:
- Regional wall motion scores.
- Global subjective assessment (eye ball technique).
- A–V plane displacement.
- ⚠ M-mode fractional shortening only measures basal function.

In systolic dysfunction, the LV is frequently dilated and valve pathology is often identified. Identifying abnormalities of diastolic function is much more complicated by echocardiography. Simple methods such as the E/A ratios on mitral pulsed-wave Doppler are confounded by age and loading conditions. Newer methods including pulmonary venous flow modalities and most recently tissue Doppler imaging provide more accurate results, which compare well with invasive haemodynamic parameters[**] (📖 Chapter 20).

Nuclear cardiology (Fig. 2.3)

Calculation of the LVEF by multiple-uptake gated acquisition scans with Technetium 99 (MUGA) or radionuclide ventriculography (RNVG) provides a more accurate and reproducible result than echocardiography.

Cardiac magnetic resonance (CMR) (Fig. 2.3)

CMR provides accurate information on LV size, volumes and LVEF. It is the most reliable non-invasive test for LVH and calculations of LV mass.

▶ CMR can be used in patients with coronary artery stents and metallic valves but not with current pacemakers/ICDs.

Angiographic LV function (Fig. 2.3)

Contrast, biplane LV angiography provides an accurate measure of LV systolic function. The gold standard of measurement of diastolic dysfunction is the assessment of pressure volumes loops during invasive haemodynamic studies.

Normal range of LVEF

LVEF is a normally distributed variable. Cut-off points for LVSD vary by the technique used, for example,
Echo LVSD   LVEF <50%.
Nuclear LVSD   LVEF <40% (differs with technique and centre).
CMR LVSD   LVEF <60%.

---

* See Leeson P et al. (2007) Echocardiography, pp. 188–95. Oxford University Press.

** See Leeson P et al. (2007) Echocardiography, pp. 198–203. Oxford University Press.

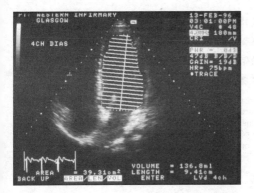

Fig. 2.2 Example of Simpson's rule for the calculation of LVEF.

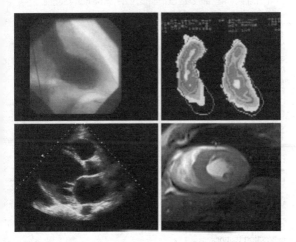

Fig. 2.3 Commonly used methods for assessing cardiac dysfunction. Top left—LV contrast angiogram. Top right—radionuclide ventriculogram/MUGA. Bottom left—2D echocardiogram. Bottom right—CMR scan. With permission from Professor Henry J Dargie.

Diagnosis of underlying aetiology of cardiac dysfunction, assessment of co-morbidities, and precipitating factors

Once the cardiac dysfunction is classified, the aetiology should be identified and, if possible, treated appropriately. Many of these tests also characterize the cardiac dysfunction more accurately and give pointers to the feasibility of future therapy. Some of the investigations also provide prognostic information, which helps to target more aggressive/invasive management (Fig. 2.4).

Commonly used tests are
- 12-lead ECG:
  - Q waves may indicate previous MI.
  - LVH may point to hypertension.
  - ST-T changes may indicate ischaemia, LVH or be non-specific.
  - QRS duration may indicate dyssynchrony.
- Exercise test:
  - This is often used to investigate underlying CHD.
  - Metabolic exercise testing is also used as a prognostic aid and to discriminate between heart and lung pathology—patients with predominant lung pathology desaturate on exercise.
- Routine blood tests (heart failure screen):
  - FBC—anaemia can be a cause or effect of HF.
  - Urea and electrolytes (Na^+, K^+).
  - Creatinine—eGFR should be estimated (📖 see Formula for estimating GFR, p. 29).
  - TFTs—hypo- and hyperthyroidism can cause HF.
  - Ferritin—haemochromatosis is a reversible cause of HF.
  - Lipids—hypercholesterolaemia is associated with the main cause of HF, ischaemic heart disease.
  - Blood glucose.
- Rarer blood tests, when aetiology is in doubt:
  - Viral titres in suspected myocarditis.
  - HIV.
  - Genetic testing (in consultation with a geneticist).
- Lung function testing:
  - FVC and FEV1 reduced in HF.
  - Reversibility testing is useful to determine future β-adrenoreceptor antagonist use.
- 24-hour Holter Monitor:
  - usually used in patients with symptomatic arrhythmias.

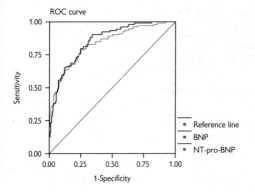

Fig. 2.4 Accuracy of BNP and NT-pro-BNP in the diagnosis of suspected heart failure. Receiver operating characteristics curves for BNP and NT-pro-BNP. Area under the curve is 0.84 (95% CI 0.79–0.89) for BNP and 0.85 (0.81– 0.90) for NTproBNP. Reproduced from Zaphiriou A. et al. *Eur J Heart Fail* 2005; **7**: 537–41 with permission from Elsevier.

Formulae for estimating GFR

MDRD-1 equation:

GFR (expressed in mL/minute/1.73m^2) = 170
 × [plasma creatinine]$^{-0.999}$ × [age]$^{-0.176}$ × [0.762 if ♀]
 × [1.180 if patient is black] × [urea]$^{-0.170}$ × [albumin]$^{+0.318}$.

MDRD-2 (abbreviated) equation:

GFR (expressed in mL/minute/1.73m^2) = 186
 × [plasma creatinine]$^{-1.154}$ × [age]$^{-0.203}$ × [0.742 if ♀]
 × [1.212 if patient is black].

Body surface area (m^2) = $\sqrt{[\text{weight (kg)} \times \text{height (cm)}/3600]}$.

Cockcroft–Gault formula for creatinine clearance (mL/minute/1.73 m^2):

♂: 1.23 × Weight (kg) × [140–age]/plasma Cr (µmol/L) × 1.73/BSA.

♀: 1.03 × Weight (kg) × [140–age]/plasma Cr (µmol/L) × 1.73/BSA.

Key reference

O'Meara E et al. The modification of diet in renal disease (MDRD) equations provide valid estimations of glomerular filtration rates in patients with advanced heart failure. *Eur J Heart Fail* 2006; **8**: 63–7.

Further echocardiography

Echocardiography can also be used to assess the following:

- Regional wall motion abnormalities suggesting CHD.
- Valve function.
- Dyssynchrony (📖 Chapter 30)[*].
- Estimation of pulmonary artery pressure.

Myocardial perfusion scanning

Planar myocardial scintigraphy or single photon emission computed tomography (SPECT) using a variety of agents (thallium, tetrafosmin, 99m technetium sestamibi) can be used to detect inducible ischaemia and hibernating myocardium.

Stress echocardiography

Echocardiography with exercise or pharmacological stress (usually with a dobutamine infusion) can be used to detect ischaemia or hibernation[**].

Coronary angiography

Invasive investigation of the coronary anatomy is indicated in patients with:

- Angina.
- Significant inducible ischaemia/hibernation on non-invasive tests.

Right and left cardiac catheterization (📖 Chapter 26)

Invasive investigation also facilitates:

- Measurement of LVEDP, PCWP, and cardiac output.
- PAP, SVR, and PVR for those where the diagnosis is in doubt, for cardiac transplantation assessment.
- Investigations of shunts with O_2-saturation data.

Cardiac biopsy (📖 Chapter 27)

This is rarely used, usually to diagnose infiltrative or inflammatory diseases such as amyloid, sarcoid, or giant cell myocarditis.

---

[*] See Leeson P et al. (2007) *Echocardiography*, pp. 463–504. Oxford University Press.

[**] See Leeson P et al. (2007) *Echocardiography*, p. 204. Oxford University Press.

Conclusions

As a result of careful assessment of the type of cardiac dysfunction, investigation of the underlying aetiology, and comorbidities, the stage should be set to

- Commence, up-titrate, and monitor general pharmacotherapy for HF.
- Identify subgroups of HF patients known to benefit from device therapy.
- Target specific therapies, such as the management of ischaemic heart disease, appropriately.
- Treat co-morbidities.
- Risk stratify those at highest risk of a poor outcome to a more advanced level of care.

Chapter 3

Estimating prognosis

Introduction

With advances in medical therapy, the prognosis of CHF has improved dramatically. However, some patients remain symptomatic and at high risk of death despite maximal medical therapy, and identifying these individuals, who would potentially benefit from a range of novel device therapies or cardiac transplantation, can be challenging.

Over 300 parameters have been shown to be predictive of a poor outcome in patients with CHF, the most consistent of which will be illustrated in this chapter. Perhaps the most promising are the B-type natriuretic peptides.

Simple clinical parameters

Demographics
Risk is greater in:
- Men.
- The elderly.
- The winter months.
- Social isolation.

Risk may fall in:
- Those with alcoholic cardiomyopathy abstaining from alcohol.

Coexisting disease
Risk is greater in patients with:
- Chronic renal failure.
- Ischaemic heart disease.
- Anaemia.
- Diabetes mellitus.
- Depression.

There is conflicting information about the prognostic role of atrial fibrillation.

Clinical parameters
Risk is greater with:
- Increasing NYHA class.
- Increasing heart rate.
- Low blood pressure.
- Low body weight (cardiac cachexia).
- Third heart sound.
- Elevated JVP.
- Syncope.
- Clinical profile—wet-cold and wet-warm at the highest risk
  (☐ see Fig. 23.3).
- Angina.
- Ventricular arrhythmias (VT/VF).

Non-invasive markers

Prognostic markers in blood tests include:
- High BNP/NT-pro-BNP (Fig. 3.1).
- Hyponatraemia.
- Increased troponin T or I.
- Anaemia.
- Increased uric acid.

Prognostic markers on ECG:
- Prolonged QRS duration (in particular LBBB).
- Ventricular arrhythmias.
- T-wave alternans—predictive of sudden death.

Prognostic markers on imaging:
- Reduced LVEF.
- Dilated LV dimensions.
- LA volume.
- Severe mitral or tricuspid regurgitation.

Markers in exercise testing:
- 6-minute walk test.
- Peak VO_2.

Invasive markers

The prognostic markers in right heart catheterization include:
- Increased pulmonary capillary wedge pressure.
- Pulmonary vascular resistance which has a linear relation to mortality and a pre-transplant PVR >3 Wood Units has been shown to increase the risk of death following surgery.

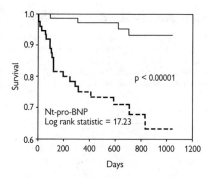

Fig. 3.1 Kaplan–Meier survival curve for NT-proBNP stratified above (broken line) and below (solid line) the median concentration, against all-cause mortality in 150 patients with advanced heart failure. Reproduced from Gardner RS et al. N-terminal brain natriuretic peptide is a more powerful predictor of mortality than endothelin-1, adrenomedullin and tumour necrosis factor-alpha in patients referred for consideration of cardiac transplantation. *Eur J Heart Fail* 2005; **7**: 253–60 with permission from Elsevier.

The heart failure survival score (HFSS)

The HFSS is a composite scoring system developed and validated in 1997. It relies on all seven clinical parameters and stratifies patients into three categories of risk: low, medium, and high (Fig. 3.2 and Table 3.1). Patients in a high-risk category, are thought to benefit from cardiac transplantation, whereas those in lower categories can be safely deferred.

Table 3.1 Heart failure survival score

Coronary artery disease (yes = 1; no = 0)	(....... × 0.6931) =	+
Intraventricular conduction delay (y = 1; n = 0)	(....... × 0.6083) =	+
Left ventricular ejection fraction (%)	(....... × –0.0464) =	+
Heart rate (bpm)	(....... × 0.0216) =	+
Na^+ concentration (mmol/L)	(....... × –0.0470) =	+
Mean arterial pressure (mmHg)	(....... × –0.0255) =	+
Peak VO_2 (mL/minute/kg)	(....... × –0.0546) =	
	HFSS =	....

- High risk   <7.19   35% 1-year survival.
- Medium risk 7.20–8.09 60% 1-year survival.
- Low risk   >8.10   88% 1-year survival.

Whilst the HFSS was developed and validated prior to the routine use of our current armamentarium of disease-modifying therapy, it has since been revalidated in more contemporary cohort. However, NT-proBNP appears to be a better prognostic marker than the HFSS in patients with advanced heart failure.

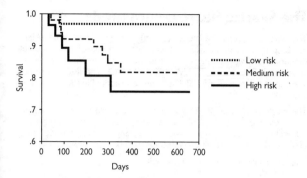

Fig. 3.2 Survival of 150 patients with advanced heart failure referred for consideration of cardiac transplantation stratified by heart failure survival score. Reproduced from Deng MC et al. Effect of receiving a heart transplant: analysis of a national cohort entered on to a waiting list, stratified by heart failure severity. Comparative Outcome and Clinical Profiles in Transplantation (COCPIT) Study Group. *BMJ* 2000; **321**: 540–5 with permission from BMJ Publishing Group Ltd.

Key references

Aaronson KD et al. Development and prospective validation of a clinical index to predict survival in ambulatory patients referred for cardiac transplant evaluation. *Circulation* 1997; 95: 2660–7.

Koelling TM, Joseph S & Aaronson KD. Heart failure survival score continues to predict clinical outcomes in patients with heart failure receiving beta-blockers. *J Heart Lung Transplant* 2004; 23: 1414–22.

Gardner RS et al. N-terminal pro-brain natriuretic peptide. A new gold standard in predicting mortality in patients with advanced heart failure. *Eur Heart J* 2003; 24: 1735–43.

PDA link: http://www.healthypalmpilot.com/cgi-bin/jump.cgi?ID=690

The Seattle heart failure model

The Seattle heart failure model (SHFM) was derived in the PRAISE-1 database of 1125 heart failure patients with the use of a multivariable Cox model. It was subsequently prospectively validated in five additional cohorts: ELITE-2, Val-HeFT, UW, RENAISSANCE, and INCHF involving 9942 heart failure patients and 17 307 person-years of follow-up (Figs. 3.3 and 3.4).

The model accurately predicts survival of heart failure patients with the use of commonly obtained clinical characteristics. Importantly, the validation cohorts included patients with a wide range of ages (14–100 years), EFs (1–75%), and heart failure symptoms (NYHA class I–IV).

The score includes the following variables:
• NYHA class.
• Ischaemic aetiology.
• Diuretic dose.
• LVEF.
• Systolic BP.
• Serum sodium.
• Haemoglobin.
• Percent lymphocytes.
• Uric acid.
• Serum cholesterol.

Renal function was not an independent predictor in this model and VO_2 was not included in the score as <1% of patients in these six data sets had this data available. Also of note is that the B-type natriuretic peptides were not included in the development of the model.

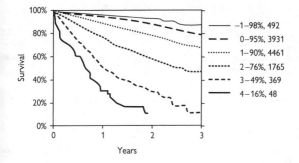

Fig. 3.3 The combined data set of the derivation and five validation cohorts for a Seattle heart failure score rounded to −1 to 4. The score, the predicted 1-year survival for the score, and the number of patients with that score are shown. Reproduced from Levy WC et al. The Seattle heart failure model: prediction of survival in heart failure. *Circulation* 2006; **113**: 1424–33 with permission from Lippincott, Williams and Wilkins.

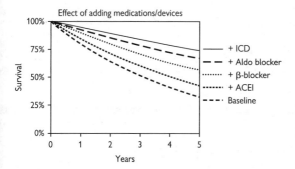

Fig. 3.4 The predicted effects on survival of sequentially adding medications and an ICD for a heart failure patient using the Seattle heart failure model. Reproduced from Levy WC et al. The Seattle heart failure model: prediction of survival in heart failure. *Circulation* 2006; **113**: 1424–33 with permission from Lippincott, Williams and Wilkins.

Key reference

Levy WC et al. The Seattle heart failure model: prediction of survival in heart failure. *Circulation* 2006; **113**: 1424–33.
PDA link: http://depts.washington.edu/shfm/SHFM.prc
Web link: www.SeattleHeartFailureModel.org

Chapter 4

Non-pharmacological management

Education

Heart failure care is becoming increasingly complex, and the patients are usually elderly. Education of patients about their condition and its management is mandatory. Careful explanation of the diagnosis and the role of each of the management choices improves adherence with therapy, where appropriate discussion may extend to end-of-life issues.

Discussion points should include:
• Diagnosis.
• Prognosis.
• Plan of investigation.
• Role of drug therapy.
• Importance of fluid management.
• Daily weight.
• Exercise training.
• Sexual activity.
• Work.
• Travel.
• Things to avoid, including smoking and excess alcohol.

The extensive range of topics to be covered highlight the value of a multi-disciplinary team approach (📖 Chapter 38). The different team members can tailor the topics to the individual patient, and their family's needs without haste and avoiding information overload at initial consultations.

If a patient is hospitalized with an episode of acute decompensated heart failure, the multi-disciplinary team should be involved in the discharge plan and follow-up.

Regular follow-up with the multidisciplinary team offers an opportunity for assessment of the development of depressive illness or stress. If depression develops and requires pharmacological intervention then the selective serotonin reuptake inhibitors are the preferred therapy.

Lifestyle modification

Unusually for cardiology there is very little prospective, randomized, controlled trial evidence to quote, when discussing advice about patient lifestyle modification. However, many of the recommendations reflect sensible health advice.

Irrespective of the aetiology of the patient's heart failure, they should be advised to:
• Stop smoking.
• Reduce alcohol consumption (<3 units/day for men and <2 units/day for women), except for alcohol-related cardiomyopathy where abstinence from alcohol should be advocated.
• In obese patients, weight loss is advised.
• Limit salt intake to <3g/day.
• Limit fluid intake to <1.5L/day if there is evidence of fluid retention. This can be relaxed to <2L/day in hot weather.

Patients should be advised to keep a daily weight chart to facilitate early detection of decompensation of their heart failure. This can be combined with advice about patient-titrated diuretic therapy. Patients are normally advised to increase their diuretic therapy by 40mg of furosemide or equivalent if the weight increases by 1kg over each of 2 consecutive days.

Exercise

A vicious cycle is established in chronic heart failure where CHF causes reduced perfusion in skeletal muscle; this triggers skeletal muscle dysfunction reducing exercise capacity. The reduced exercise capacity further deconditions the patient, worsening the heart failure and so the skeletal muscle hypoperfusion.

There is a convincing body of evidence that exercise training in heart failure improves symptoms and quality of life (Fig. 4.1). There is some evidence from meta-analyses that it may even reduce hospitalization and improve survival, and this has led the National Institutes for Health in the USA to sponsor the HF-ACTION trial to look in detail at the efficacy and safety of exercise training in heart failure.

The ACC/AHA guideline recommends exercise training, in conjunction with pharmacological therapy, in patients with reduced LVEF and CHF. Current evidence advocates the use of exercise training in stable NYHA II or NYHA III heart failure.

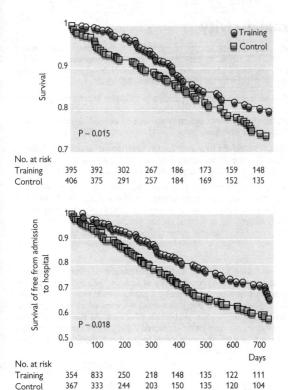

Fig. 4.1 Kaplan-Meier plots of cumulative 2-year survival (top) and 2-year survival free from hospitalization (bottom) in a meta-analysis of patients with CHF involved in exercise training and controls. Reproduced from Piepoli MF *et al.* Exercise training meta-analysis of trials in patients with chronic heart failure (ExTraMATCH). BMJ 2004; **328**: 189 with permission from BMJ Publishing Group Ltd.

Key reference
Gottlieb SS *et al.* Effects of exercise training on peak performance and quality of life in congestive heart failure patients. *J Card Fail* 1999; **5**: 188–94.

Sexual activity

Patients may express anxiety about sexual activity after a diagnosis of heart failure is made. In patients with stable, compensated NYHA I–II heart failure, sexual activity is considered safe. NYHA III–IV suggests that symptoms of heart failure may preclude sexual activity.

In ischaemic cardiomyopathy, patients with angina should be advised to avoid sexual activity that induces chest pain and reminded that the use of nitrates absolutely contraindicates the use of sildenafil and other phosphodiesterase-5 inhibitors.

The use of β-blockers may increase the likelihood of impotence. Referral to a specialist impotence clinic may be appropriate as there are many pharmacological and non-pharmacological aids that may be of benefit.

Hypertrophic cardiomyopathy is a specific condition that requires risk stratification before advising the patient about sexual activity. An exercise test and echocardiogram are useful in risk stratification because of the possibility of syncope or sudden cardiac death related to exertion. If this suggests high risk, then the patient should be advised to defer sexual activity until appropriate intervention is complete (myomectomy, septal ablation ± ICD).

Patients with an ICD or CRT-D implanted should be aware of the small risk of device activation related to sexual activity. They should be advised that their partner would not receive a painful shock. However the partner may be aware of the shock or a muscle spasm, which while startling, will not be painful! Normal post-shock advice should then be instituted with emergency services being contacted if the patient remains unstable. If the patient is well, the local cardiology service should be contacted within 24 hours for a device check.

Employment

As part of the assessment of a patient with CHF, it is important to address their employment status. If their job is predominantly sedentary, then it should be possible to continue despite their diagnosis. Physical jobs may require review and support in considering alternative employment.

If the severity of symptoms precludes full-time employment, then the multidisciplinary team may be able to assist in negotiating reduced hours, retraining or identifying relevant social security benefits.

Travel advice

Patients with stable, compensated heart failure may be reassured about their safety to travel. However, they should be advised to ensure that they have adequate medical cover included in their travel insurance and that the insurance company is aware of their diagnosis. General travel advice should include carrying a full supply of medication for the trip in original containers with a list of medications in their hand luggage.

The mode of travel should be considered. Travel by car will allow route planning to facilitate the needs of a diuretic user. They should be encouraged to stop every 2–3 hours and mobilize to reduce development of dependent oedema and deep venous thrombosis. Rail travel makes these considerations easier to accommodate.

Passengers using air travel should be similarly advised. The additional considerations for flights include whether oxygen will be required (☐ see p. 52 for guidelines). A further issue for an increasing number of patients with CHF is that they may have an implantable device that could trigger airport security systems. They should carry their device card with them at all times and present it to the security staff. A manual search is then performed.

Immunization

CHF is associated with pulmonary oedema and pulmonary hypertension. These increase the risk of developing pulmonary infection that is poorly tolerated because of the cardiac co-morbidity. Immunizing CHF patients against influenza has been shown to reduce hospitalization for decompensated heart failure by 37%.

It is advised that patients with CHF should receive
• Pneumococcal vaccine.
• Annual influenza immunization.

Nutrition

As detailed in (☐ Chapter 19), there are specific cardiomyopathies that result from nutritional deficiencies, for example, beri beri (vitamin B_1/thiamine). Dietary advice is obviously crucial in the management of these patients.

All patients with CHF could benefit from nutritional advice in terms of nutritional balance, calorie restriction in the obese, and nutritional supplementation in cardiac cachexia.

Oxygen and aviation

Air travel has become a routine feature of life. The diagnosis of CHF may indicate that the patient is more at risk from reduced oxygen tension as found in commercial aircraft.

The British Thoracic Society guidelines for oxygen on commercial airlines suggests using pulse oximetry on room air at sea-level, as a screening test:
- pO_2 > 95% suggests that oxygen will not be required.
- pO_2 < 92% suggests that oxygen will be required.

For patients with a pO_2 between 92–95% on room air at sea level, the presence of CHF requires that hypoxia testing be performed, with a 15min challenge of an FiO_2 of 15%. The results are interpreted as follows:
- pO_2 >7.4 kPa (>55mmHg)   In-flight oxygen not required
- pO_2 6.6–7.4 kPa (50–55mmHg)   Borderline. A walk test may be helpful
- pO_2 <6.6 kPa (<50mmHg)   In-flight oxygen (2L/min)

▶▶ Particular caution must be applied in the assessment of patients with CHF due to congenital heart disease.

Key references

British Thoracic Society Recommendations. British Thoracic Society Standards of Care Committee. Managing Passengers with Respiratory Disease Planning Air Travel http://www.brit-thoracic.org.uk/c2/uploads/FlightRevision04.pdf (accessed June 2007)

Mortazavi A et al. Altitude-related hypoxia: risk assessment and management for passengers on commerical aircraft. Aviat Space Environ Med 2003; 74: 922–7.

Chapter 5

Pharmacological management

The key drugs

The medical treatment of heart failure has been revolutionized by large randomized, controlled clinical trials studying the effects of antagonists of the renin–angiotensin–aldosterone and sympathetic nervous systems. These drugs now form the cornerstone in the management of the condition.

The individual pharmacology and evidence for use of specific drugs is covered in Chapters 31–7. For drugs to avoid in patients with HF, (🕮 see Chapter 4).

Angiotensin converting enzyme inhibitors (ACEi) (🕮 see also Chapter 31)

- These are first-line agents for all patients with heart failure due to left ventricular systolic dysfunction (LVSD)—this is also true in patients with asymptomatic LVSD.
- Unless there is a contraindication, their use should be considered mandatory.
- They unequivocally reduce both morbidity and mortality in clinical trials with an average relative risk reduction of 20–5%.
- Use with caution in patients with significant renal disease (see Table 5.1).
- Angioedema with previous use is an absolute contraindication.
- Drugs with proven efficacy in clinical trials are captopril, enalapril, ramipril, lisinopril, trandolapril (see Table 5.1).

How to use ACE inhibitors in clinical practice (see opposite)

- ACE inhibitors can usually be safely started in the outpatient setting.
- Start at a low dose and up-titrate at weekly/fortnightly intervals as blood pressure and renal function allow and no symptoms of hypotension.
- It is advisable to stop potassium-sparing diuretics prior to commencement of ACEi.
- Often, in elderly or frail patients, stopping the loop diuretic facilitates the introduction.
- Check renal function within 1 week.
- Beware of hyperkalaemia.
- Watch for ACEi induced cough (5–10%).
- Use with caution in aortic stenosis.
- Symptomatic hypotension can be minimized by nocturnal dosing.

Table 5.1 ACE inhibtors with an evidence base in LVSD and their suggested dosing

Drug	Start dose (mg)	Target dose (mg)	Frequency
Captopril	6.25	50–100	tds
Enalapril	2.5	10–20	bd
Ramipril	1.25	5	bd
Trandolapril	0.5	4	od
Lisinopril	2.5	30–35	od

Worsening renal function

- Some increase in urea, creatinine, and potassium is to be expected after initiation of an ACE inhibitor; if an increase is small and asymptomatic no action is necessary.
- An increase in creatinine of up to 50% above baseline, or 266μmol/L (3mg/dL), whichever is the smaller, is acceptable.
- An increase in potassium to a value <5.5mmol/L is acceptable.
- If urea, creatinine, or potassium do increase excessively, consider stopping concomitant nephrotoxic drugs (e.g. NSAIDs), other potassium supplements/retaining agents and, if no signs of congestion, reducing the dose of diuretic.
- If greater increases in creatinine or potassium than those outlined above persist despite adjustment of concomitant medication, the dose of the ACE inhibitor should be halved and blood chemistry rechecked within 1–2 weeks; if there is still an unsatisfactory response, specialist advice should be sought.
- If potassium increases to >5.5mmol/L or creatinine increases by >100% or to above 310μmol/L (3.5mg/dL) the ACE inhibitor should be stopped and specialist advice sought.
- Blood chemistry should be monitored frequently and serially until potassium and creatinine have plateaued.

Adapted from McMurray J et al. Eur J Heart Fail 2005; **7**: 710–21 with permission from Elsevier.

β-adrenoceptor antagonists (📖 see also Chapter 32)

- These are also mandatory drugs for all patients with heart failure due to LVSD (this is also true in patients with asymptomatic LVSD post-myocardial infarction).
- They unequivocally reduce both morbidity and mortality in clinical trials with a 35% relative risk-reduction on average.
- They can be used in patients with COPD but are contra-indicated in patients with significant reversal airways obstruction (check pulmonary function tests).
- Peripheral vascular disease is not a contra-indication to β-adrenoceptor antagonist therapy.
- Drugs with proven efficacy in clinical trials are carvedilol, bisoprolol, metoprolol CR/XL, and nebivolol (see Table 5.2).

How to use β-adrenoceptor antagonists in clinical practice

- Can be initiated safely in the outpatient setting.
- In patients with more advanced disease, or those who are elderly/frail, inpatient commencement should be considered.
- Start at a low dose and up-titrate every 2–4 weeks, provided pulse >50/minute and systolic BP >90mmHg.
- Use with caution in first-degree heart block.
- Contra-indicated in higher degrees of heart block.
- Do not commence in decompensated heart failure (e.g. in patients with pulmonary or peripheral oedema, or in the ITU setting on inotropes).
- Titrate to the maximum tolerated dose (📖 see Chapter 32).
- In patients on β-adrenoceptor antagonists admitted with decompensated heart failure, continue current dose if possible, or reduce one dose decrement. Only stop the β-adrenoceptor antagonist if absolutely necessary.

Table 5.2 β-adrenoreceptor antagonists with an evidence base in CHF and their suggested dosing

Drug	Start dose (mg)	Up-titration steps (mg)	Target dose (mg)	Frequency
Carvedilol	3.125	6.25–12.5 to 25–50*	25/50*	bd
Bisoprolol	1.25	2.5–5 to 7.5–10	10	od
Metoprolol CR/XL	12.5[†]/25	25–50 to 100–200	200	od
Nebivolol	1.25	2.5–5 to 10	10	od

* In patients over 85kg.
[†] In patients in NYHA class III/IV.

Aldosterone antagonists (📖 see also Chapter 33)
- These are reserved for NYHA III/IV patients with CHF due to LVSD.
- They reduce both morbidity and mortality in clinical trials by 30%.
- The drug with proven efficacy is spironolactone (and eplerenone in post-MI HF/LVSD and diabetes).

How to use spironolactone in clinical practice
- Use with caution if the baseline creatinine is >221µmol/L.
- Monitor within 1 week after starting for renal dysfunction and hyperkalaemia.
- Use with caution in the elderly.
- Stop spironolactone temporarily during episodes of diarrhoea and/or vomiting.
- Men may experience painful gynaecomastia; in these cases, eplerenone can be substituted.

Angiotensin receptor antagonists (ARB) (📖 see also Chapter 34)
- These can be used in patients with ACEi intolerance due to cough or due to angioedema; they produce similar reductions in cardiovascular endpoints to ACEi.
- They cause similar amounts of renal dysfunction as ACEi.
- Again, start at low dose and up-titrate checking renal function and blood pressure.
- Drugs with proven efficacy are: losartan, valsartan, and candesartan.
- Candesartan and valsartan can also be added to ACEi in patients who remain symptomatic.

Diuretics (📖 see also Chapter 35)
- In general, this is loop diuretic therapy, that is, furosemide, bumetamide, or torasemide.
- These are for relief of symptoms and signs of pulmonary or peripheral congestion.
- Use the minimum dose necessary to render the patient euvolaemic.
- Side-effects to look out for are renal dysfunction, hypokalaemia, hyponatraemia, hyperglycaemia, and gout—that is monitor U&E's.
- Rather than increasing to industrial doses (i.e. >80mg bd furosemide or equivalent), add a thiazide diuretic (e.g. bendrofluazide 2.5mg) or metolazone (2.5–5mg) to block differing sites in the nephron and overcome diuretic resistance
- With the above strategy, monitor U&Es carefully.
- Remember to advise patients to adhere to a fluid restriction (📖 Chapter 4).
- Patients should be encouraged to tailor their diuretic therapy according to weight and needs.

General principles for use of key drugs

- Clearly there are many drugs to be introduced.
- Remember to seek specialist advice, especially in patients with more advanced heart failure or more complex drug regimens.
- It is better to achieve small doses of ACEi and β-adrenoreceptor, rather than a larger dose of either alone.
- Optimum pharmacological therapy is best achieved within a multi-disciplinary management programme, where up-titration and monitoring can be rigorously adhered to (see Section VI).
- Particularly with combinations of disease-modifying therapy, careful monitoring of renal function should be undertaken.
- The flow diagram of pharmacotherapy is summarized in Fig. 5.1.

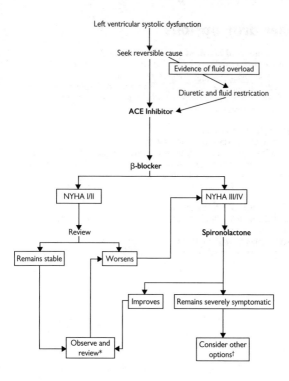

Fig. 5.1 Flow diagram of pharmacological therapy for CHF according to patient status.

*Review process:
- Symptoms
- Signs
- Weight
- U&Es

- Can disease modifying therapy be optimized? Angiotensin receptor antagonists are now indicated, in addition to angiotensin converting enzyme inhibitors and β-blockers, in NYHA II patients
- Can diuretics be reduced?

†Consider:
- Digoxin
- Increasing diuretic if evidence of cardiac decompensation
- Biventricular pacing
- Cardiac transplanation
- Anticoagulation in atrial fibrillation, LV thrombus

Other drug options

Hydralazine and nitrates (see also Chapter 37)
- Consider using this in the case of patients intolerant to both ACE-inhibitors and angiotensin receptor antagonists.
- Consider this as an additional agent to standard medical therapy for CHF (ACE/ARB plus β-blocker and/or aldosterone antagonists) in African-Americans.

Digoxin (see also Chapter 36)
- The role of digoxin appears less clear.
- Introduce digoxin in patients who remain symptomatic, for example with frequent hospitalizations despite maximal medical therapy, or to provide rate control to patients with atrial fibrillation (AF).
- It should be avoided in those with ventricular arrhythmias.

Anti-platelet and anticoagulants
- Patients with IHD should be on aspirin unless there is a specific contra-indication.
- The benefits of warfarin therapy in CHF are currently uncertain, except in patients with atrial fibrillation or known LV thrombus.

Drugs to use with caution or avoid

Non-steroidal anti-inflammatory drugs (NSAIDs) are associated with deterioration of heart failure symptoms by systemic vasoconstriction. They do not in themselves cause heart failure. They may also cause renal dysfunction and exacerbate renal dysfunction associated with ACE inhibitors, angiotensin receptor blockers, or aldosterone antagonists.

Corticosteroids should be prescribed with care, as the balance between beneficial effects and detrimental effects in terms of fluid balance needs to be established.

Calcium channel blockers, except amlodipine and felodipine, are negatively inotropic and can be associated with decompensation of heart failure and increased mortality. Amlodipine or felodipine may be used in patients with CHF and poorly controlled angina or hypertension. Patients should be advised of the higher incidence of pulmonary and leg oedema associated with amlodipine.

The use of carvedilol, bisoprolol, and metoprolol CR/XL in the management of left ventricular systolic dysfunction is well established. β-**blockers with intrinsic sympathomimetic activity** (e.g. pindolol and acebutolol) should be avoided as they can cause deterioration in heart failure status.

The majority of **anti-arrhythmic drugs** have negatively inotropic effects and can cause a deterioration in heart failure. The pro-arrhythmic nature of heart failure is exacerbated by some of the anti-arrhythmics, particularly those with class I actions (e.g. flecainide). In supraventricular arrhythmias, sinus rhythm may be maintained using amiodarone or dofetilide (not licensed for use in the UK). Consideration should be made of the possibility of radio-frequency ablation to cure the dysrhythmia. If atrial fibrillation is the accepted rhythm, then rate control can usually be achieved by one of the accepted β-blockers and with digoxin if required. Ventricular arrhythmias often require an ICD. Further rhythm control to reduce events may be achieved with beta-blockade or amiodarone.

Cilostazol is licensed for the treatment of intermittent claudication. It is a phosphodiesterase inhibitor that has arterial vasodilator effects. Based on studies of other phosphodiesterase inhibitors that have demonstrated increased mortality in CHF, the FDA have advised that cilostazol should not be prescribed to any patient with a diagnosis of heart failure.

The oral hypoglycaemic agents **metformin** and **thiazolidinediones** (e.g. rosiglitazone and pioglitazone) should be used with caution in patients with CHF. Metformin is associated with a risk of lactic acidosis that can be life threatening. The FDA guidance is that metformin should not be used in patients with CHF requiring pharmacological therapy. Many practitioners use metformin with caution in patients with CHF and only withhold it during acute decompensated episodes or if renal failure or liver failure occurs. The thiazolidinediones cause fluid retention and should, therefore, be avoided in patients with decompensated CHF, and stopped if fluid retention occurs.

Phosphodiesterase-5 inhibitors such as sildenafil are established treatments for erectile dysfunction in men. They can cause systemic hypotension and are therefore are contraindicated if the patient is taking any nitrate preparation or an α-blocker. A small study of sildenafil in men with NYHA II or III CHF suggested that the reduction in blood pressure was small (6mmHg) and asymptomatic.

Patients with CHF should be advised to abstain from **illicit drugs** including cocaine and amphetamines which may cause an acute decompensation of their heart failure symptoms. Caution should be advised in the use of **homeopathic remedies** particularly those with catecholeamine-like actions (ma huang, ephedra, and ephedrine and its metabolites). Other natural remedies may have significant interactions with anticoagulants (e.g. St John's wort, *Gingko biloba*, ginseng and homeopathic garlic), digoxin (e.g. hawthorne and St John's wort), β-blockers, vasodilators, and anti-arrhythmics.

α-Adrenoreceptor antagonists (e.g. doxazosin and prazosin) have no role in the treatment of HF and may exacerbate it.

Chapter 6

Device therapy in CHF

Introduction

The majority of patients with heart failure stabilize or improve with pharmacological therapy. Device therapy in heart failure addresses two potential consequences of left ventricular dysfunction, namely malignant ventricular arrhythmias that can lead to sudden cardiac death (SCD) and ventricular dyssynchrony. These two phenomena can coexist in the CHF patient. Implantable cardiac defibrillators address the issue of SCD and cardiac resynchronization therapy is aimed at those with dyssynchrony.

Cardiac resynchronization therapy pacing (CRT-P), also known as multi-site pacing or biventricular pacing, has a clear role in selected patients with advanced heart failure who remain symptomatic despite maximum tolerated pharmacological therapy. Implantable cardiac defibrillators (ICD) have also been shown to reduce arrhythmic deaths in both ischaemic and non-ischaemic cardiomyopathy. CRT-P can be combined with ICD functions (CRT-D) to achieve the benefits of both devices.

The implantation of any of these devices carries with it the usual risks associated with pacemaker implantation: infection and lead displacement being the most common; and also the need for regular hospital contact; and ultimately, generator change. While the risk of complications is relatively low, mainly causing minor inconvenience, it does highlight the importance of appropriate patient and device selection. Up to 50% of shocks delivered by ICDs may be inappropriate, again, stressing the importance of patient selection.

Dual chamber pacing in CHF

Standard dual chamber pacing was investigated as a potential therapeutic intervention that might facilitate
• More aggressive use of beta-blockers.
• Optimization of atrioventricular delay, reducing mitral regurgitation.

The DAVID study compared VVI pacing (lower rate limit of 40bpm) with DDDR pacing (lower rate limit of 70bpm) after implantation of an ICD. At the time of data analysis it was realized that the DDDR group had been paced 60% of the time whilst the VVI group were only paced 1% of the time. Thus, the study demonstrates the effect of DDDR pacing compared to sinus rhythm. A significantly higher number of patients died or were hospitalized with heart failure in the group who were DDDR paced (27%, versus 16% in the VVI group). Such pacing is thought to induce mechanical dyssynchrony by effectively causing LBBB. Therefore, standard dual chamber pacing is not recommended as a therapy for heart failure.

In patients who require pacing for the treatment of bradycardia, consideration should be made as to whether they qualify for CRT. If not, then dual chamber pacing should be used as backup only with pacing algorithms set to minimize paced beats. Trials are currently underway to compare CRT with DDDR pacing for bradycardia pacing in heart failure patients.

Key reference

Wilkoff BL *et al.* Dual-chamber pacing or ventricular backup pacing in patients with an implantable defibrillator: the Dual Chamber and VVI Implantable Defibrillator (DAVID) Trial. *JAMA* 2002; **288**: 3115–23.

Dyssynchrony

Cardiac resynchronization therapy aims to address the problem of ventricular dyssynchrony in heart failure. Dyssynchrony is a complex phenomenon (Fig. 6.1). It can be thought of as occurring at three levels: electrical, structural, and mechanical. These levels are, of course, interrelated.

- *Electrical dyssynchrony* consists of inter- or intraventricular conduction delay.
  - Usually electrical dyssynchrony manifests as a left bundle branch block (LBBB).
  - LBBB occurs in 24% of patients with LV systolic dysfunction.
  - It becomes more common as the severity of the LVD increases (38% of patients with moderate to severe CHF).
  - The mortality of CHF increases in proportion to the QRS width.
- *Structural dyssynchrony* results from the disruption of the myocardial collagen matrix impairing electrical conduction and mechanical efficiency.
- *Mechanical dyssynchrony* manifests as regional wall motion abnormalities leading to:
  - Increased workload and stress.
  - Paradoxical septal wall motion.
  - Presystolic mitral regurgitation.
  - Reduced diastolic filling times.

These features of dyssynchrony further exacerbate systolic dysfunction. Atrioventricular conduction delay that often occurs in heart failure is also associated with features that adversely affect systolic function:

- Loss of 'top up' from atrial systole at the end of ventricular diastole. In atrial fibrillation this has been shown to reduce cardiac output by 25–40%.
- Atrioventricular delay results in delayed closure of the mitral valve with resultant mitral regurgitation.

The subject is made more complicated by the observation that not all patients with LBBB have evidence of mechanical ventricular dyssynchrony and a small proportion of patients with a normal QRS duration do have echocardiographic evidence of dyssynchrony.

LBBB or intraventricular conduction delays that result in ventricular dyssynchrony can be reversed by pacing both ventricles. Cardiac resynchronization therapy (CRT) can also address the atrio-ventricular conduction delay that often occurs in heart failure.

(a)

(b)

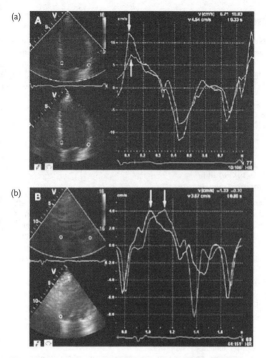

Fig. 6.1 (See colour plate 1) Colour-coded tissue Doppler images, four-chamber
views. Left ventricular dyssynchrony is defined as the delay in peak systolic
velocities between the basal septum and the basal lateral wall.
(a). Tracings from a normal individual. The arrows indicate the peak systolic
velocities, illustrating perfect synchrony between the two walls.
(b). Tracings showing extensive left-ventricular dyssynchrony in a patient with
severe heart failure. The arrows indicate the peak systolic velocity in each curve,
illustrating dyssynchrony of 130ms duration. The tissue Doppler tracings are
obtained from samples placed in the basal part of the septum (yellow curve) and
the lateral wall (green curve). Reproduced from Bleeker GB et al. Left ventricular
dyssynchrony in patients with heart failure: pathophysiology, diagnosis and
treatment *Nat Clin Pract Cardiovasc Med* 2006; **3**: 213–19 with permission from
Nature Publishing Group.

Cardiac resynchronization therapy

CRT-P typically uses leads in the right atrium, right-ventricular apex and the coronary sinus. The coronary sinus lead paces the left ventricular free wall.

CRT-P has been shown to improve
• Quality of life.
• Left-ventricular ejection fraction.
• Exercise capacity.
• Contractile function.
• Reverse LV remodelling.

CRT-P has been shown to reduce
• Hospital admissions.
• Mortality in NYHA III/IV.
• Pulmonary capillary wedge pressure.

All these changes in haemodynamics result in improved myocardial efficiency and reduced myocardial oxygen demand. After implantation of CRT-P, cessation of resynchronization for only 72 hours results in marked deterioration of rate of rise of left-ventricular systolic pressure and mitral regurgitation. For maximal effects to be obtained, biventricular pacing should be achieved >85% of the time.

Indications
Current guidelines require patients to fulfil all of the following criteria:
• NYHA III or IV heart failure despite stable, optimal medical therapy.
• LVEF <35%.
• Sinus rhythm.
• Electrical dyssynchrony—QRS duration >150ms or 120–149ms if evidence of mechanical dyssynchrony.

These criteria derive from the landmark clinical trials that established the morbidity and mortality benefits of CRT-P (COMPANION and CARE-HF) (Table 6.1). However, approximately one-third of patients have been reported not to improve with CRT-P (non-responders). In an attempt to identify these patients it has been suggested that *mechanical* dyssynchrony should be proven on echocardiography before implanting the CRT-P device. In CARE-HF, patients with QRS duration between 120 and 150ms were required to have two out of three echocardiographic measures of dyssynchrony. Patients with QRS >150ms could proceed directly to CRT. (Chapter 30 on dyssynchrony.)

Patients with mechanical dyssynchrony who have a narrow QRS may benefit from CRT-P. However, to date, there are no large-scale, prospective, randomized trials that demonstrate that CRT-P based solely on the assessment of mechanical dyssynchrony improves clinical outcomes.

Table 6.1 Trials of CRT-P ± D and CHF

	No. of patients	LVEF (%)	Follow-up (months)	Key finding
MUSTIC (2001)	67	23	3	CRT-P improved 6 MWT
MIRACLE (2002)	453	24	6	CRT-D improved QoL, NYHA, and 6 MWT
PATH-CHF (2002)	42	21	12	No difference between CRT and LV pacing
CONTAK-CD (2003)	490	21	6	CRT-P improved peak VO_2 and 6 MWT
MIRACLE-ICD (2003)	369	24	6	CRT-D improved QoL, NYHA and peak VO_2
PATH-CHF II (2003)	101	23	3	CRT-P in QRS duration >150ms improved peak VO_2, 6 MWT, and QoL
COMPANION (2004)	1520	22	17	CRT-P and CRT-D reduced time to death and CHF hospitalization; CRT-D also reduced all cause mortality
CARE-HF (2005)	813	26	29	CRT-P reduced all cause mortality, improved LVEF, and QoL

Key trial

CARE-HF—The effect of cardiac resynchronization on morbidity and mortality in heart failure.
  Design: RCT of CRT versus standard medical therapy.
  Subjects: n = 813; NYHA III/IV; LVEF ≤35%; mean age = 67 years; 74% 4; median QRS
      duration = 160ms; median LVEF = 25%.
  Follow up: 1.9 years.
  Results: 37% RRR in mortality or CV hospitalization (p < 0.001).
      36% RRR in mortality (p < 0.002).
      6.9% absolute increase in LVEF after 18 months (p < 0.001).
      1122pg/mL fall in NT-proBNP after 18 months (p < 0.002).
      Improvement in quality of life (p < 0.001).
  Reference: Cleland JG et al. The effect of cardiac resynchronization on morbidity and morality
      in heart failure. N Engl J Med 2005; **352**: 1539–49.

Although the criteria for the trials include QRS duration >120ms, the majority of patients included in the trials had a wide LBBB morphology. The mean QRS direction in CARE-HF was 160ms. The efficacy of CRT-P in RBBB is not established but the inclusion criteria are based on QRS duration not morphology.

▶ It must be stressed that the benefits seen in the large outcome trials of CRT were in addition to optimal pharmacological therapy, that is, ACE inhibition, β-blockade, and aldosterone antagonism

CRT-P in atrial fibrillation

Patients with atrial arrhythmias were excluded from CARE-HF. The MUSTIC-AF trial is a small trial that compared RV pacing with biventricular pacing in patients with heart failure, a wide QRS, and chronic AF who required a pacemaker for bradycardia. Only 37 patients completed the crossover phase, limiting the interpretation of the trial, however significant improvements were seen in exercise capacity. This is not sufficient evidence to advocate the use of CRT-P in these patients. However, in patients with chronic AF and heart failure who require AV nodal ablation for arrhythmia control, biventricular pacing appears to be better than standard pacing.

Key reference

Leclercq C et al. Comparative effects of permanent biventricular and right-univentricular pacing in heart failure pacing in chronic atrial fibrillation. *Eur Heart J* 2002; **23**: 1780–7.

Optimization of CRT

There are aspects of CRT that must be addressed in order to optimize pacing in an individual. These relate to the positioning of the LV lead and then optimization of the pacing settings of the AV delay and VV interval.

Ventricular pacing position

The LV lead should be positioned on the free wall of the LV at the point of latest activation. In general, this is on the postero-lateral or postero-inferior wall of the LV—achieved by positioning the LV lead in the marginal cardiac vein or postero-lateral cardiac vein. This is not always possible as it is determined by cardiac venous anatomy. In ischaemic cardiomyopathy, LV lead placement should avoid regions of infarction scar.

After the LV lead is positioned, the RV lead can be positioned to maximize the distance between them and so optimize the effect of the resynchronization. Usually, the best position for the RV lead is the RV apex.

Atrioventricular delay

There are two potential benefits in optimizing AV delay—reduced mitral regurgitation and improved left-ventricular diastolic filling time, with resultant improvement in cardiac output.

Atrioventricular delay delay optimization protocols use Doppler echocardiography. These can either measure LV diastolic filling time (mitral inflow) or LV systolic function (aortic VTI). Aortic VTI has been suggested to achieve a greater increase in stroke volume.

Mitral inflow method

Pulsed-wave transmitral velocities are measured at the mitral leaflet tips. Diastolic filling time is the time from onset of transmitral flow to closure of the mitral valve. The rationale is to maximize the distance between the E and the A waves without the A wave being truncated by mitral-valve closure.

The AV delay is determined by the time between ventricular activation and the end of the A wave at an AV delay of 160ms (*a*). LV electromechanical delay is the time from LV stimulation to closure of the mitral valve (*b*). The optimized AV delay is then set as (160 − (*b*–*a*)) ms (see Fig. 6.2).

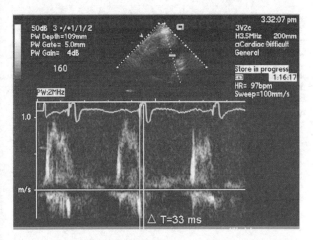

Fig. 6.2 Doppler signals for mitral inflow method. Reproduced from Kerlan JE *et al*. Prospective comparison of echocardiographic atrioventricular delay optimisation methods for cardiac resynchronization therapy. *Heart Rhythm* 2006; **3**: 148–54 with permission from Elsevier.

Aortic VTI method

Continuous-wave Doppler from an apical five-chamber window is used to measure the aortic VTI. Whilst pacing in VDD mode the AV delay is decreased from 200ms to a minimum of 60ms in 20ms increments. After at least 10 paced beats at the pacing interval, a mean of 3 beats is taken to establish the aortic VTI. The AV delay is then fine tuned in 10ms increments. The optimized AV delay is the one that results in the maximum aortic VTI (Fig. 6.3).

V–V interval

No long-term data are available to suggest that altering the VV interval improves outcome in CRT-P. However, small studies do suggest that altering the VV pacing interval can affect surrogate measure of cardiac output such as the echocardiographic aortic VTI. The VV interval has to be individually optimized as some patients respond to pacing the RV first, some others to pacing the LV first, and yet others benefit from simultaneous RV and LV pacing.

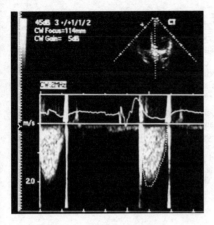

Fig. 6.3 Doppler signals for aortic VTI method. Reproduced from Kerlan JE *et al*. Prospective comparison of echocardiographic atrioventricular delay optimization methods for cardiac resynchronization therapy. *Heart Rhythm* 2006; **3**: 148–54 with permission from Elsevier.

Follow up of the patient post-CRT

It is important to remember that the patient post-CRT still has heart failure. They should be followed up, preferably in a heart failure clinic. Specifically, patients who respond to CRT often have an immediate increase in their cardiac output and blood pressure. This can result in an improvement in renal function. Patients should therefore be seen at 1-week post-CRT to ascertain whether they require a reduction in their diuretic therapy.

Thereafter, due consideration should be given to optimizing their heart failure therapy. Specifically, this should include up-titration of the β-blocker dose, which may have been previously hampered by bradycardia. In addition, it may be possible to up-titrate doses of ACEI or ARB if CRT has improved arterial blood pressure and/or renal function. Addition of spironolactone may also be feasible in some patients post-CRT, where it proved difficult beforehand. To derive maximum benefit, ideally, patients post-CRT should be cared for within a multi-professional heart failure programme.

Implantable cardiac defibrillators

Heart failure is an arrhythmogenic condition arising from a combination of structural heart disease and electrolyte imbalance. Further pro-arrhythmic stress occurs in ischaemic cardiomyopathy due to ischaemic events. Ventricular arrhythmias, from premature ventricular beats through to ventricular fibrillation, occur in >80% of patients with heart failure and cardiomyopathy. Up to 50% of heart failure deaths are sudden cardiac death (SCD)—usually arrhythmic. However, the proportion of patients dying suddenly in heart failure decreases with increasing severity of the condition. Trials of specific pharmacological anti-arrhythmic therapy for the prevention of SCD have been disappointing.

Implantable cardiac defibrillators have revolutionized the management of arrhythmias. An implantable cardiac defibrillator (ICD) is an advanced form of pacemaker that can detect and treat arrhythmias—usually ventricular arrhythmias. Several types of system are available—a single bipolar lead placed in the right-ventricular apex, a dual chamber device with an atrial lead to improve distinction of atrial from ventricular arrhythmias, or an ICD can be combined with CRT-P, so-called CRT-D.

Most ICDs use heart rate criteria to determine VT and VF. This can be important, particularly, in young patients who may achieve sinus tachycardia into the arrhythmia detection zone, or patients with fast paroxysmal atrial arrhythmias. ICDs use the following detection qualifiers to distinguish VT and VF:
- Rate detection zone.
- Detection cycles: the number of consecutive beats required to diagnose arrhythmia.
- Rate stability: VT is a relatively stable rhythm, so this feature establishes the maximum inter-beat variation that still allows VT to be diagnosed.
- Sudden onset: ventricular arrhythmias usually have a sudden onset compared to sinus tachycardia that gradually ramps up.

ICD therapies may offer shock therapy only or be programmable allowing attempts at overdrive (anti-tachycardia) pacing of VT before resorting to defibrillation. Tiered therapy allows increasingly aggressive therapy in the treatment of VT that is likely to be haemodynamically stable, usually defined as a heart rate of 200bpm or cycle length of 300ms (Table 6.2). This cut-off may be inappropriate in patients with heart failure who are less likely to tolerate fast arrhythmias. An important part of ICD implantation is fine-tuning of the device to meet the individual patient's requirements.

Table 6.2 Conversion of heart rate in beats/minute into R–R interval (cycle length) in milliseconds

R–R interval = 1000/(HR/60)									
HR (bpm)	300	290	280	270	260	250	240	230	220	210
R–R (ms)	200	207	214	222	231	240	250	261	273	286
HR (bpm)	200	190	180	170	160	150	140	130	120	110
R–R (ms)	300	316	333	353	375	400	429	462	500	545
HR (bpm)	100	90	80	70	60	50	40	30	20	10
R–R (ms)	600	667	750	857	1000	1200	1500	2000	3000	6000

▶▶ **Magnet mode in ICDs**

Placing and keeping a magnet over the ICD deactivates the defibrillator—useful if recurrent inappropriate shocks.

Indications for ICD therapy

The indications for ICD therapy in heart failure have emerged from the publication of several large RCTs (Tables 6.3–6.5). The MADIT II study showed a mortality benefit for ICDs in patients with IHD who had a LVEF <30%. Notably, this was a study conducted with patients with LVD who did not necessarily have heart failure. More recently, the SCD-HeFT study was carried out on patients with CHF in NYHA II and III with LVEF <35%, of either ischaemic or non-ischaemic aetiology. The study showed a reduction in all-cause mortality for those treated with ICDs (particularly in NYHA II) compared to those on optimal medical therapy or optimal medical treatment plus amiodarone, that is, amiodarone did not confer any survival benefit.

NICE guidelines suggest that ICDs should not be used in patients with NYHA IV heart failure.

They should be used for:

Secondary prevention of SCD in the following cases
- Survivors of sudden cardiac death (excluding those with acute myocardial infarction or reversible cause).
- Sustained ventricular tachycardia causing syncope or haemodynamic compromise.
- Sustained ventricular tachycardia without syncope/cardiac arrest, with LVEF <35% and NYHA I-III heart failure.

Primary prevention of SCD in non-ischaemic cardiomyopathy
- LVEF <35% and NYHA II-III.

Primary prevention of SCD in ischaemic cardiomyopathy
- History of previous MI (>40 days previous) and both the following:
  - LVEF <30%.
  - Non-sustained VT on Holter monitoring.

Some guidelines also advocate the demonstration of inducible VT at electrophysiological testing.

The implementation of these guidelines could have huge resource implications. To try to identify patients who do not need an ICD there are numerous studies ongoing. Currently, one of the most promising techniques is microvolt T-wave alternans (MTWA). A recent study showed that compared to patients with a negative MTWA test, patients with ischaemic cardiomyopathy and a positive MTWA test had more than double the risk of
- All cause mortality.
- Arrhythmic mortality.

Table 6.3 Primary prevention trials of ICD and ischaemic cardiomyopathy

	No. of patients	LVEF (%)	Follow-up (months)	Mortality (%)		
				Control	ICD	p value
MADIT (1996)	196	26	27	39	16	0.0009
CABG-Patch (1997)	900	27	32	21	22	0.64
MADIT II (2002)	1232	23	20	20	14	0.007
DINAMIT (2004)	674		30	17	19	0.66
SCD-HeFT (2005)	2521	25	45.5	29	22	0.007

Table 6.4 Secondary prevention trials of ICD and ischaemic cardiomyopathy

	No. of patients	LVEF (%)	Follow-up (months)	Mortality (%)		
				Control	ICD	p value
AVID (1997)	1016	35	18	24	16	0.02
CIDS (2000)	659	34	35	30	25	0.14

Table 6.5 Primary prevention trials of ICD and non-ischaemic cardiomyopathy

	No. of patients	LVEF (%)	Follow-up (months)	Mortality (%)		
				Control	ICD	p value
CAT (2002)	104	24	27	31	26	0.55
AMIOVERT (2002)	103	22	32	13	12	0.80
DEFINITE (2004)	450	21	20	14	9	0.06
SCD-HeFT (2005)	2521	25	45.5	29	22	0.007

Key reference

Chow T et al. Prognostic utility of microvolt T-wave alternans in risk stratification of patients with ischemic cardiomyopathy. J Am Coll Cardiol 2006; **47**: 1820–7.

Contraindications
- Reversible cause for VT or VF.
- Co-morbidity limiting prognosis.
- Patient choice.

In ischaemic cardiomyopathy, there is currently no evidence for implantation in the first month post-MI. The DINAMIT study demonstrated no difference in outcome in those treated with an ICD or medical therapy. There was a trend towards harm early on for the ICD group.

ICDs are used in addition to optimal medical therapy. In order to reduce the frequency of ICD events, β-blocker therapy should be maximized where possible.

Healthcare providers must be considerate in supporting patients in whom ICDs are to be implanted as many may struggle with the concept. Also the patient should be advised as to what to do and who to contact if the device is activated.

Key references

A comparison of antiarrhythmic-drug therapy with implantable defibrillators in patients resuscitated from near-fatal ventricular arrhythmias. The Antiarrhythmics versus Implantable Defibrillators (**AVID**) Investigators. *N Engl J Med* 1997; **337**: 1576–83.

Bardy GH *et al.* Amiodarone or implantable cardioverter-defibrillator for congestive heart failure (**SCD-HeFT**). *N Engl J Med* 2005; **352**: 225–37.

Hohnloser SH *et al.* Prophylactic use of an implantable cardioverter-defibrillator after acute myocardial infarction (**DINAMIT**). *N Engl J Med* 2004; **351**: 2481–8.

Kadish A *et al.* Prophylactic defibrillator implantation in patients with nonischaemic dilated cardiomyopathy (**DEFINITE**). *N Engl J Med* 2004; **350**: 2151–8.

Lee DS *et al.* Effectiveness of implantable defibrillators for preventing arrhythmic events and death: a meta-analysis. *J Am Coll Cardiol* 2003; **41**: 1573.

Moss AJ *et al.* Prophylactic implantation of a defibrillator in patients with myocardial infarction and reduced ejection fraction (**MADIT-II**). *N Engl J Med* 2002; **346**: 877–83.

Combination of CRT with ICD—CRT-D

Deciding whether to implant CRT-P or CRT-D is difficult and requires, at this time, a consideration of both the CRT and ICD evidence as only one trial has addressed the use of CRT-D in heart failure.

The COMPANION trial demonstrated that patients with a QRS duration >120ms with NYHA III-IV heart failure, nearly half of whom had non-ischaemic cardiomyopathy, had a survival benefit from CRT-D compared optimal medical therapy. Patients with CRT-P had a trend towards a reduction in all-cause mortality. The difference between CRT-P and CRT-D in the trial was not statistically significant. Both CRT-D and CRT-P significantly reduced the primary endpoint in this study—that of all cause mortality or admission to hospital with heart failure. The mortality benefit from CRT-D begins immediately after implantation, but CRT-P seems to require reverse remodelling to take place before mortality benefit is seen.

In addition, many of the patients included in CARE-HF would now meet the criteria for an ICD based on their LVEF and NYHA class. As sudden cardiac death is more common in NYHA II heart failure than in NYHA III (64% versus 33%), theoretically, if CRT-P improves NYHA class for those in class III, it may, in fact, increase the likelihood of sudden cardiac death by moving them into stage II! For this reason, in future, the majority of devices implanted in patients with heart failure are likely to be CRT-D. However in the short-term, because of financial considerations in socialized health care systems, the majority of devices implanted will be CRT-P.

Key reference

Bristow MR et al. Cardiac-resynchronization therapy with or without an implantable defibrillator in advanced chronic heart failure (**COMPANION**). N Engl J Med 2004; **350**: 2140–50.

Which device in whom?

Symptomatic CHF

On the basis of current trial evidence, the following device management is suggested for the patient in sinus rhythm. However, the cost implications of this strategy are huge, and the reality is that local guidelines should be followed.

NYHA I	No device
NYHA II or III **and** QRSd <120ms	Consider ICD
NYHA III or IV **and** QRSd 120–149ms	Echo to assess for dyssynchrony: Present—consider CRT-P or -D (if NYHA III) Absent—consider ICD (if NYHA III)
NYHA III **and** QRSd >150ms	Consider CRT-P or -D
NYHA IV **and** QRSd >150ms	Consider CRT-P

▶ If implanting non-CRT devices, aim for a minimum amount of ventricular pacing.

Asymptomatic LVSD

The device management of asymptomatic LVSD is more difficult. By definition, these patients are in NYHA class I. Therefore, the only trial evidence that is available is from the post-myocardial infarction populations studied in MADIT I and MADIT II, and MUSTT. In the non-ischaemic population with LVSD, SCD-HeFT considered patients in NYHA II or III and DEFINITE was not significant in its findings and suggested a trend that benefit was only seen in the symptomatic patients.

In the post-myocardial infarction population with ischaemic cardiomyopathy and an LVEF <30%, the MADIT II data suggests survival benefit with the implantation of an ICD.

Again, this has to be assessed at local level and often on an individual patient basis as the cost ramifications of such a policy is significant.

There is no evidence-base at present to suggest that there is a role for CRT in the asymptomatic population.

Implantable haemodynamic monitoring devices

Device therapy, including cardiac resynchronization therapy and implantable cardiac defibrillators, is becoming an important part of the heart failure treatment of an increasing proportion of patients with CHF. These devices can be combined with haemodynamic monitoring sensors. The haemodynamic parameters available include:
- Pulmonary artery pressure—sensor in the pulmonary artery.
- Right ventricular pressure—sensor in RV.
- SVO_2—oxygen saturation sensor in the RV.
- Electrogram—distal tip electrode in RV lead.
- Intrathoracic impedance—from RV tip to device.

From the data collected, it is possible to estimate RV dP/dt_{max}. This is derived from the observation that the right-ventricular dP/dt_{max} occurs as the pulmonary valve opens and the RV and PA pressures equilibrate. The RV dP/dt_{max} estimates the PA diastolic pressure.

The electrogram allows determination of rhythm (for example, to calculate the burden of atrial fibrillation), heart rate, and heart rate variability. These data, combined with a trace of activity level, can identify deterioration in the patient's cardiac status which is likely to result in hospitalization: the heart rate rises as the heart rate variability and activity level fall. Intrathoracic impedance is inversely correlated with PCWP. It is sensitive to the fluid content of the lung parenchyma. Thus, if fluid begins to accumulate in the lungs the intrathoracic impedance falls. This change happens before patient symptoms develop.

The COMPASS-HF trial demonstrated a reduction in hospitalization in the NYHA III subgroup in a RCT of an implantable pulmonary artery pressure device versus usual care. Currently, there are several ongoing trials of invasive monitoring devices. By the early identification of deterioration in fluid status, it is hoped that proactive therapy can be instituted to improve their volume status and hopefully prevent the need for hospital admission. This is an attractive alternative to the current situation where the majority of diuretic manipulation is in reaction to symptomatic deterioration.

The stage beyond isolated information from invasive monitors is the integration of this data with non-invasive measures, such as weight and blood pressure, and correlation with patient symptoms. Technology is now available that achieves all of this and can relay this information to the patient's physician via the telephone or Internet. Thus, without leaving their home the patient can benefit from regular follow-up. Such technology challenges clinicians to ensure robust arrangements are in place so that all of the information is logged and action taken where necessary.

Key references

Adamson PB et al. Continuous autonomic assessment in patients with symptomatic heart failure: prognostic value of heart rate variability measured by an implanted cardiac resynchronization device. *Circulation* 2004; **110**: 2389–94.

Yu CM et al. Intrathoracic impedance monitoring in patients with heart failure: correlation with fluid status and feasibility of early warning preceding hospitalization. *Circulation* 2005; **112**: 841–8.

Coronary revascularization in heart failure

Introduction

Ischaemic heart disease is the most common cause of heart failure in westernized countries. It is important to identify these patients for two reasons:

- The potential for revascularization with improvement in left ventricular systolic function and mortality.
- The survival of patients with ischaemic cardiomyopathy is poorer than those with non-ischaemic aetiology.

Ischaemic cardiomyopathy involves two distinct pathological processes; **myocardial infarction** with irreversible damage and **myocardial ischaemia**. The latter can have an impact on LV dysfunction in three ways:

- *Inducible ischaemia* can lead to a transitory reduction in LV performance.
- *Hibernating myocardium* that can have contractility restored with revascularization.
- *Stunned myocardium* describing a more transient contractile dysfunction secondary to an ischaemic insult.

Diagnosis of ischaemic cardiomyopathy

As described in Chapter 2, heart failure is not a diagnosis and the aetiology should be found. The rigour with which the diagnosis of IHD is sought varies from centre to centre. Some perform diagnostic coronary angiography in all HF subjects, whereas others restrict the procedure to those with chest pain or evidence of ischaemia on non-invasive testing (exercise testing or myocardial perfusion imaging). The latter approach is often applied in those with comorbidities which may increase the complication rate of angiography.

What is to be done, in terms of revascularization in the patient with IHD and no chest pain, remains controversial and will only be resolved once large outcome trials randomizing patients to revascularization (CABG and/or PCI) with optimal medical therapy report.

Management of the patient with chest pain and HF is less contentious. Data exists from older trials, for example, CASS suggesting that revascularization by CABG results in a survival benefit for those with severe coronary artery disease and LV dysfunction.

Once the diagnosis of IHD has been confirmed, it is reasonable to assess myocardial viability.

Assessment of myocardial viability

While coronary angiography details coronary anatomy it does not provide information about the myocardial perfusion. The optimal method to assess for viability remains contentious. Few studies have been performed that directly compare all the techniques in the same patient population. In addition, there are new techniques in development that may offer more detailed evaluation of hibernating myocardium, one of the most promising is stress perfusion cardiac magnetic resonance (CMR) imaging. Among all patients with ischaemic cardiomyopathy, 20–50% have a significant burden of hibernating myocardium.

The predictive accuracy of the tests for assessing for myocardial viability is illustrated in Fig. 7.1. The choice of test depends on local availability and expertise. Myocardial perfusion imaging is more sensitive but dobutamine stress echo is more specific in predicting the likelihood of improvement of left-ventricular systolic function after revascularization.

Caution should be applied when assessing the myocardial viability scans, as the techniques depend on comparative blood flow, so 'balanced ischaemia' which can occur with, e.g. left main-stem stenosis, can mask severe ischaemia with potentially extensive areas of viable myocardium.

Tests for assessing myocardial viability
- Myocardial perfusion imaging.
  - Thallium stress-redistribution-reinjection SPECT.
  - Thallium stress rest-redistribution SPECT.
  - Technetium-sestamibi SPECT.
- Stress CMR.
- FDG-positron emission tomography scanning.
- Echocardiography.
  - Dobutamine stress.
  - Myocardial contrast.

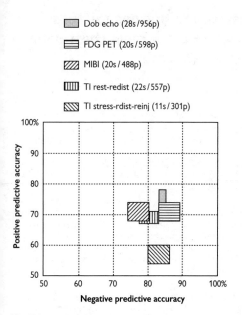

Fig. 7.1 Weighted mean positive and negative predictive accuracy of the different imaging tests for predicting recovery of segmental function after revascularization from a meta-analysis of patients with ischaemic LV dysfunction. The rectangles are centered on the weighted means and the size of the rectangles indicates 95% confidence intervals. The number of averaged studies (s) and patients (p) for each technique is indicated. Reproduced from Underwood SR et al. *Eur Heart J* 2004; **25**: 815–36 with permission from Oxford University Press.

Revascularization options for those with IHD who do not have chest pain or inducible ischaemia

Several prospective randomized, controlled studies are ongoing to determine whether revascularization, either percutaneous or surgical, improves outcome in such patients. These include the STICH trial looking at surgical intervention, and the HEART-UK and PARR-2 trials (PCI and/or CABG).

While the outcome of these trials is awaited, observational studies suggest a survival advantage in patients with ischaemic cardiomyopathy with viable myocardium undergoing coronary artery bypass grafting (CABG) compared to medical therapy (annual mortality 3.2% versus 16%). Following CABG, the LVEF improved by a mean of 8% but this improvement can take weeks to months to occur.

The role of percutaneous intervention with coronary angioplasty is less well established. It is an attractive option, as it would remove the necessity of the patient undergoing major surgery. Observational studies are difficult to interpret because patients undergoing PCI and not CABG have often been declined surgery because of severity of disease or comorbidity. A registry comparing patients with ischaemic cardiomyopathy undergoing PCI with a historical control group suggests that PCI reduced mortality, MI, and need for CABG.

At present, guidelines from the ACC/AHA suggest that in ischaemic cardiomyopathy CABG should only be offered to asymptomatic patients with

- Proven significant regions of hibernating myocardium.
- Left main stem stenosis.
- Left main equivalent (proximal LAD and Cx stenoses).
- Proximal LAD stenosis with two or three vessel disease.

A significantly dilated LV (LVEDD >7cm) carries a high operative mortality (Fig. 7.2).

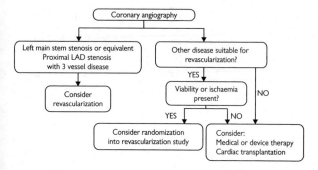

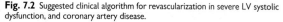

Fig. 7.2 Suggested clinical algorithm for revascularization in severe LV systolic dysfunction, and coronary artery disease.

Key references

Allman KC et al. Myocardial viability testing and impact of revascularisation on prognosis in patients with coronary artery disease and left ventricular dysfunction: a meta-analysis. *J Am Coll Cardiol* 2002; **39**: 1151–8.

Holper EM et al. The impact of ejection fraction on outcomes after percutaneous coronary intervention in patients with congestive heart failure: an analysis of the NHLBI Percutaneous Transluminal Coronary Angioplasty Registry and Dynamic Registry. *Am J Cardiol* 2006; **151**: 69–75.

Chapter 8

Other surgical techniques

Introduction

Other surgical options in the treatment of chronic heart failure include left-ventricular assist devices—LVADs (as a bridge to transplantation, a bridge to recovery, or as destination therapy), ventricular remodelling, mitral valve repair, and revascularization for hibernating myocardium.

The option of surgical intervention is at times overlooked in caring for a patient with heart failure. If, in spite of maximal tolerated medical therapy, the patient continues to deteriorate then referral for consideration of cardiac transplantation may be appropriate. However, as the algorithm given in the opposite page illustrates (Fig. 8.1), other surgical techniques may be considered earlier in the course of management for a range of heart failure aetiologies. The role of some of the newer techniques continues to evolve.

 This is currently an area with a paucity of RCT evidence.

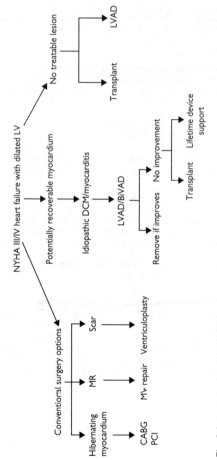

Fig. 8.1 Surgical options in heart failure

Mitral valve surgery

Functional mitral regurgitation from loss of leaflet co-aptation is a frequent complication of end-stage heart failure, due to ventricular and thus mitral annular dilatation, and is associated with a poorer survival. Thus, mitral valve repair has been established to benefit ambulant patients with severe heart failure and mitral regurgitation. The operative mortality is approximately 5%, but patients often improve symptomatically enough to drop several NYHA classes.

Mitral valve repair is an operation that preserves the sub-valvular apparatus and aims to restore the valve function by improving the valve geometry. One option for repair is to use an 'edge-to-edge' approximation of the anterior and posterior leaflets in their mid-portion with suture plication—the Alfieri repair. However, a much more commonly performed procedure is an annular ring, either partial around the posterior aspect of the annulus or complete around the entire annulus, which may enhance the resulting morphology. Mitral valve repair is often better tolerated than replacement. The adequacy of repair is assessed in theatre with intra-operative TOE. The long-term results are unknown as it has never been subject to a RCT.

In heart failure with ischaemic aetiology, mitral valve surgery may be combined with coronary artery bypass surgery or surgical remodelling of the left ventricle (e.g. DOR procedure). A surgical ablation procedure of the atria (e.g. MAZE) may be performed in association with the mitral valve repair, to treat or prevent atrial fibrillation.

Contra-indications to mitral valve repair
- Primary mitral valve dysfunction
- More than mild aortic regurgitation

Mitral valve replacement in heart failure also results in a fully competent valve, but also in altered LV geometry post-operatively, and this can have disastrous effects on the patient. The left ventricle, which had been failing pre-operatively despite the low resistance offered by the incompetent mitral valve, often deteriorates rapidly as it struggles to adapt to the post-operative volume demands and altered geometry. Therefore, mitral valve replacement is not routinely recommended for the treatment of mitral incompetence in patients with heart failure.

Key reference

Wu AH *et al.* Impact of mitral valve annuloplasty on mortality risk in patients with mitral regurgitation and left ventricular systolic dysfunction. *J Am Coll Cardiol* 2005; **45**: 381–7.

Left-ventricular reconstruction surgery

Following a myocardial infarction, the diseased area of myocardium undergoes necrosis, followed by fibrotic change and ultimately the production of scar tissue. Non-damaged areas of myocardium become hypertrophied to compensate for the lack of contractility of the infarcted area, and eventually become dilated. Left-ventricular remodelling occurs when segments of viable muscle dilate remote from scar, resulting in volume enlargement and geometric distortion. By removing dyskinetic segments, and so reducing the left-ventricular dimensions, the law of Laplace predicts a reduction in wall stress. Various surgical techniques have been performed to remove aneurysmal myocardium, with the ultimate aim of improving left-ventricular function. Left-ventricular aneurysmectomy has a recognized role in the treatment of heart failure, both to improve symptoms and reduce the risk of ventricular arrhythmias. However, surgical ventricular remodelling, without revascularization awaits results of clinical trials.

▶ LV aneurysmectomy is indicated in patients with large, discrete left ventricular aneurysms who develop heart failure.

Cooley first described left-ventricular reconstruction surgery in 1958. The technique was modified by Jatene in 1985, and again in 1989 by Dor. The SAVER (surgical anterior ventricular endocardial restoration) procedure is a further modification of the Dor procedure that excludes non-contracting anterior wall segments in the dilated left ventricle following anterior myocardial infarction.

Dilated cardiomyopathies are associated with global left-ventricular dilatation. Batista developed the partial left ventriculectomy in 1996 to reduce wall stress and so improve left-ventricular function. It has not become routine because of high operative mortality and uncertain long-term survival. Late scar-related ventricular arrhythmias required the implantation of prophylactic implantable defibrillators.

The modern left-ventricular reconstruction operations result in improved LVEF and NYHA functional class, and may have a favourable effect on mid-term mortality. They can be combined with coronary artery revascularization surgery and carry a low operative mortality of 3%.

Key references

Dor V et al. Left ventricular aneurysm: a new surgical approach. *Thorac Cardiovasc Surg* 1989; **37**: 11–9.

Elefteriades JA et al. Left ventricular aneurysmectomy in advanced left ventricular dysfunction. *Cardiol Clin* 1995; **13**: 59–72.

Menicanti L & Di Donato M. The Dor procedure: what has changed after fifteen years of clinical practice? *J Thoracic Cardiovasc Surg* 2002; **124**: 886–90.

Passive cardiac restraint

Progressive left-ventricular dilatation has been shown to be an independent marker of death and adverse outcome in patients with heart failure. In 1985, Carpentier and Chachques described cardiomyoplasty, which wrapped *latissimus dorsi* around the heart and used electrical stimulation to augment left-ventricular function. The technique is no longer in clinical use because of detrimental outcomes in the limited number of patients studied.

However, the cardiomyoplasty technique did demonstrate that providing a 'girdle effect' to the left ventricle reduced progressive enlargement by reducing wall stress. The ACORN CorCap is a polyester sock that provides passive cardiac restraint. Initial studies suggest improved symptoms with its use, but these studies were not powered to assess the effect of the device on mortality. To date, no cases of constrictive physiology have been reported, and this is thought to be because the atria are carefully excluded from the device when it is applied. Further studies of this device are in progress.

Key reference

Konertz WF et al. Passive containment and reverse remodelling by a novel textile cardiac support device. *Circulation* 2001; **104**: 1270.

Mechanical cardiac support (1)

In CHF, mechanical cardiac support may be required as a short-term therapy to support recovery during acute decompensation. Alternatively, mechanical support may be a medium-term option to stabilize a patient to allow time for myocardial recovery (e.g. in fulminant viral myocarditis) or for a heart to become available for cardiac transplantation. Finally, mechanical support may be accepted as definitive therapy in place of cardiac transplantation in patients with contraindications to transplantation.

In non-ischaemic cardiomyopathies, the haemodynamic effects of mechanical cardiac support result in reverse remodelling of the myocardium. This includes:
- Increased contractile strength.
- Structural remodelling with restoration of ventricular geometry and cytoskeletal proteins, and reduced myocardial fibrosis and hypertrophy of cardiomyocytes.
- Improved neurohormonal profile including reversal of the downregulation of β-adrenoceptors.

These processes occur surprisingly quickly and studies suggest that they are essentially complete by 40 days after initiation of mechanical support. In one study comparing the exercise capacity of patients following implantation of a left-ventricular assist device with cardiac transplant recipients, the peak VO_2 at 12 weeks in the LVAD group was comparable to that of the transplant cohort at 12 weeks and 1 year.

Mechanical cardiac support covers a spectrum of techniques that can be classified as follows:
- Extracorporeal ventricular support—*short-term*
  - IABP (📖 see Chapters 24 and 28)
  - Pulsatile ventricular assist device (VAD)
  - Non-pulsatile VAD
- Extracorporeal membrane oxygenation—*short-term*
- Intracorporeal ventricular support
  - Pulsatile left ventricular assist device (LVAD)
  - Total artificial heart
- Intracorporeal ventricular assist devices
  - Non-pulsatile LVAD

The short-term strategies used in acute heart failure and acute decompensated chronic heart failure are discussed in 📖 Chapter 24.

Complications of the mechanical cardiac support devices
- Haemolysis with resulting need for transfusion, which is a concern in pre-transplantation patients.
- Thromboembolism including cerebrovascular events, therefore anticoagulation is essential.
- Bleeding.
- Device-related infection.
- Mechanical dysfunction or failure.

Key references

de Jonge N et al. Exercise performance in patients with end-stage heart failure after implantation of a left ventricular assist device and after heart transplantation: an outlook for permanent assisting? *J Am Coll Cardiol* 2001; **37**: 1794–9.

Vatta M et al. Molecular remodelling of dystrophin in patients with end-stage cardiomyopathies and reversal in patients on assistance-device therapy. *Lancet* 2002; **359**: 936–41.

Mechanical cardiac support (2)

There are more than 40 different devices currently available or in trial stages. These are some of the more widely studied devices.

Thoratec ventricular assist device
This is the currently the most widely used device in North American practice. It can act as a right ventricular assist device (RVAD), left ventricular assist device (LVAD), or biventricular assist device (BiVAD). The atria are cannulated with outflow into the appropriate artery (i.e. pulmonary artery or aorta). The suction pump for each ventricle is outside the body. The result is pulsatile flow.

Jarvik 2000 pump
This axial-flow impellar pump provides continuous rather than pulsatile flow. It is small and is completely implantable. The other novel feature of this device is that the powerline is tunnelled subcutaneously and exits the skin at the base of the skull. This location is based on the observation that patients with cochlear implants are not troubled by infection at their percutaneous exit site.

Thoratec HeartMate LVAD
There are two versions of this device: pneumatic and vented-electric. Both have percutaneous drivelines. The LVAD connects the apex to the ascending aorta through a sub-diaphragmatic drive pump. The major attraction of this device is that anticoagulation is not required but is generally advised. This has been achieved by the development of a tex-tured polyurcthane inner surface that becomes coated with a protein layer.

Baxter Novacor
This device propels blood from the left-ventricular apex to the ascending aorta. An electromagnet triggers a pusher plate, collapsing a bladder that forces blood from the apex to the aorta, through two valves that prevent regurgitation. Unfortunately, this device is particularly prone to throm-boembolic complications even in the presence of full anticoagulation.

Total artificial heart
These devices are inserted into the thorax in place of the patient's ventricles taking blood from the atria with outflow into the pulmonary artery and aorta. It is currently used as a bridge to transplantation. There are percutaneous drivelines, which unfortunately act as a potential inlet for infection. The device in clinical use is the CardioWest pneumatic total artificial heart (TAH). In one study comparing implantation of the CardioWest TAH with optimal medical therapy, those receiving the TAH had a higher rate of survival to transplantation and survival to 1 year.

Screening scale prior to insertion of LVAD

This score was developed from patients receiving the HeartMate LVAD.
(From: Rao V et al. Revised screening scale to predict survival after insertion of left ventricular assist device. *J Thorac Cardiovasc Surg* 2003; **125**: 855–62.)

- Ventilator support   *4 points*
- Postcardiotomy shock   *2 points*
- Temporary LVAD prior to Heart Mate implant   *2 points*
- Central venous pressure >16mmHg   *1 point*
- Prothrombin time >16 seconds   *1 point*

The points are added together to give a risk score (Table 8.1).

Table 8.1 Risk score

Risk	Points	Operative mortality (%)	Successful bridge to transplantation (%)
Low	0–4	8	89
Intermediate	5–7	32	65
High	8–10	49	49

Key references

Morgan JA et al. Bridging to transplant with the HeartMate left ventricular assist device: The Columbia Presbyterian 12-year experience. *J Thoracic Cardiovasc Surg* 2004; **127**: 1309–16.

Rao V et al. Revised screening scale to predict survival after insertion of left ventricular assist device. *J Thoracic Cardiovasc Surg* 2003; **125**: 855–62.

Mechanical cardiac support (3)

Mechanical cardiac support and cardiac transplantation

The timing of transplantation has been demonstrated to be very important in outcome of patients receiving mechanical support devices. As stated previously, mechanical support improves survival to transplantation and reduces post-transplantation mortality.

An analysis of 466 patients who had received cardiac transplants after LVAD support demonstrated that those who received a transplant within 2 weeks of LVAD implant had a 1-year survival of 74%, whilst those who received their transplant more than 6 months after LVAD implant had a 1-year survival of 76%. By contrast, those who had a transplant 4–6 weeks after LVAD implantation had a 1-year survival of 92%.

The LVAD requires a window of time to facilitate resolution of end-organ dysfunction, particularly renal failure. However, beyond 6 months complications from the LVAD, particularly thromboembolic and septic events begin to impact on transplantation success.

Bridge to recovery—when to withdraw support?

The use of mechanical cardiac support to bridge to recovery has required an assessment of how to assess when to withdraw support. In one series of 131 patients with dilated cardiomyopathy, 24% (32 patients) of devices were withdrawn without transplantation. Those who had successful withdrawal and persistent recovery had recovered an LVEF ≤45% and LVEDD ≤55mm.

In a separate study of 111 patients, successful explantation of the device could be considered in those with an exercise capacity allowing a peak VO_2 of greater than 20mL/kg/minutes and/or a peak cardiac output of >10L/minutes. This achieved successful explantation of the LVAD in only five patients in their study group.

Trials are ongoing to establish the optimal pharmacological combination for use with LVAD support. A recent study used bisoprolol, a specific β_1 adrenoreceptor blocker, and then added clenbuterol, a specific β_2 adrenoreceptor agonist, when LV remodelling was established in a small study of highly selected patients with non-ischaemic cardiomyopathy. With this regime 11 of 15 patients successfully bridged to recovery and explantation of the LVAD.

Key references

Birks EJ et al. Left ventricular assist device and drug therapy for the reversal of heart failure. *N Engl J Med* 2006; **355**: 1873–84.

Burkhoff D, Klotz S & Mancini DM LVAD-induced reverse remodelling: basic and clinical implications for myocardial recovery. *J Card Fail* 2006; **12**: 227–39.

Dandel M et al. Long-term results in patients with idiopathic dilated cardiomyopathy after weaning from left ventricular assist devices. *Circulation* 2005; **112**: 137–45.

Gammie JS et al. Optimal timing of cardiac transplantation after ventricular assist device implantation. *J Thorac Cardiovasc Surg* 2004; **127**: 1789–99.

Mancini DM et al. Low incidence of myocardial recovery after left ventricular assist device implantation in patients with chronic heart failure. *Circulation* 1998; **98**: 2383–9.

Mechanical cardiac support (4)

Mechanical cardiac support as destination therapy

To date, one randomized, controlled trial has been carried out in patients with advanced heart failure who are ineligible for cardiac transplantation, namely, REMATCH. The trial included 129 patients in NYHA class IV heart failure. They were randomized to receive either the LVAD, or to optimal medical therapy. The primary endpoint of the trial was death from any cause. There was a reduction of 48% in the risk of death from any cause in the group receiving the LVAD: the relative risk was 0.52 (95% CI 0.34–0.78), a significant difference with a p value of 0.001. However, although mortality was statistically reduced, few patients in the group that received the assist device survived longer than 2 years and there were significant limitations with the device used, including infection, bleeding, and device failure. This trial has resulted in the FDA approving LVADs as destination therapy in USA. However, other countries are awaiting further trials with newer devices before committing to such an expensive therapy for heart failure.

Key reference

Rose EA *et al.* Longterm mechanical left ventricular assistance for end-stage heart failure. *N Engl J Med* 2001; **345**: 1435–43.

Chapter 9

Cardiac transplantation

Introduction

Cardiac transplantation (CTx) is the final option for patients who remain symptomatic despite optimal medical and device therapy. However, while the patient's condition should be sufficiently severe to justify this procedure, he or she should also be free of significant comorbidities so that major cardiac surgery and the ensuing immunosuppressive regime can be tolerated by him or her.

Christian Barnard performed the first human–human heart transplant in 1967 in South Africa. CTx was revolutionized in 1976 with the discovery of cyclosporin A, which dramatically improved patient survival.

- Annually, there are approximately 3000 cardiac transplantations performed worldwide.
- CTx remains a low-volume procedure with 45% of institutions averaging <10/year and 77% of institutions <20/year.
- The primary indication for CTx worldwide is equally balanced between heart failure of an ischaemic aetiology and dilated cardiomyopathy, each accounting for approximately 45%.
- The average age of the CTx recipient is 51.9 (±11.6) years compared to that of the donor of 33.4 (±13.1) years, and over three-quarters (77.6%) of recipients are male, compared with two-thirds of donors.

Indications for referral

- Advanced CHF refractory to maximum tolerated medical therapy or surgical therapy: patients who benefit have an expected annual mortality rate in excess of 25%, and their limiting symptoms should be predominantly attributable to heart failure.
- Life-threatening acute heart failure unresponsive to initial therapy (e.g. post-MI cardiogenic shock).
- Refractory life-threatening arrhythmias.
- Intractable angina not amenable to revascularization or other methods of pain control.

Contra-indications

Absolute contra-indications
- Irreversible pulmonary hypertension (see p. 126).
- Advanced irreversible hepatic disease.
- Irreversible pulmonary parenchymal disease, for example, FEV1 <50% predicted.
- Cerebrovascular disease not amenable to revascularization.
- Active infection.
- Life expectancy markedly compromised by other systemic disease.
  - For example, amyloid*, sarcoid, and vasculitides.
- Inability to comply with medical therapy/immunosuppressive regime.
- Continuing alcohol- or substance-misuse.

Relative contra-indications
- Age >70 years.
- Advanced irreversible renal disease (eGFR <40mL/min).
- Diabetes mellitus with end-organ damage.
- Peripheral vascular disease not amenable to revascularization.
- Malignancy: collaborate with oncologists to establish risk stratification.
- Hepatitis B, C, or HIV positive.
- Severe obesity (BMI >30).
- Recent pulmonary embolism, that is, within 3 months.
- Active peptic ulcer disease.
- Severe osteoporosis.
- Smoking.
- Learning disability/dementia.

* The exception to this is amyloid if it is predominantly affecting the heart (on SAP scans) and the underlying plasma cell dyscrasia is eradicated by chemotherapy or transplantation.

Key reference
Mehra MR *et al*. Listing criteria for heart transplantation: International Society for Heart and Lung Transplantation guidelines for the care of cardiac transplant candidates. *J Heart Lung Transplant* 2006; **25**: 1024–42.

Patient selection

- The selection of patients for CTx is difficult and traditionally involves clinical assessment and an assimilation of markers of the severity of CHF such as the LVEF and peak VO_2.
- The recommended investigations for CTx assessment are shown in (Table 9.1).
- It is important to identify those patients at the highest risk of mortality prior to listing, as CTx is far from a benign surgical procedure, with a 1-year mortality of approximately 19% (Fig. 9.1).
- The assessment process also attempts to rule out the presence of any significant contra-indication.
- A panel-reactive antibody >10% requires prospective lymphocyte crossmatch.

How to assess reversibility of pulmonary hypertension

Irreversible pulmonary hypertension is an absolute contra-indication to CTx. It is defined as follows:
- Pulmonary vascular resistance (PVR) >5 Wood units, or
- PVR index (PVRI) >6, or
- Transpulmonary gradient (TPG) >16mmHg, or
- PA systolic >60mmHg + one of the three criteria listed in the bullet points above.

If PVR 2.5–5, reversibility should be assessed as follows:
- The Swan–Ganz catheter should remain *in situ*.
- Give oxygen therapy.
- Infuse a vasodilator whilst maintaining systolic blood pressure >85mmHg.
- If unsuccessful, an infusion of dobutamine can be tried.

If PVR is reversed, then the regime should be recorded in the notes. The PVR should be checked every 6 months.

If the PVR can be reduced to <2.5 but the systolic BP is <85mmHg, the patient remains at high risk of RV failure and death, following CTx.

How to assess reversibility of GFR <40mL/min:
- Give IV dobutamine for 48 hours.
- Commence at 2.5µg/kg/min.
- Increase as tolerated (heart rate and rhythm, BP).
- Repeat GFR.

If repeat GFR is >40mL/min, it suggests that the impairment is cardiac-pump related and should improve following CTx.

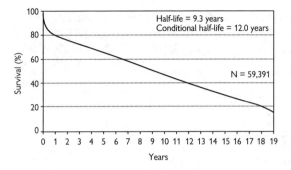

Fig. 9.1 Actuarial survival for heart transplants performed between January 1982 and June 2001. Conditional half-life is the time to 50% survival for those recipients surviving the first year post-transplantation. Reproduced from Taylor DO *et al.* The registry of the International Society for Heart and Lung Transplantation: twentieth official adult heart transplant report—2003. *J Heart Lung Transplant* 2003; **22**: 616–24 with permission from Elsevier.

Trans-pulmonary gradient (TPG) = Mean PAP–PCWP.
PVR = TPG/cardiac output (measured in Wood units).

> **Example**
> Normal TPG approximately 6mmHg.
> Normal cardiac output (CO) approximately 5L/minute.
>
>   PVR = 6/5 = 1.2 Wood units.

1 Wood unit = 80 dyne s/cm^5.
Normal range for pulmonary vascular resistance = 1.25–2.5 Wood units.
Normal range for pulmonary vascular resistance = 100–200 dyne s/cm^5.

   Body surface area = square root of ((height (cm)
                        × weight (kg)/3600).

   PVR index (PVRI) = PVR/body surface area.

Table 9.1 Recommended schedule for heart transplant evaluation

Test	Baseline	Repeat 3 months	Repeat 6 months	Repeat 9 months	Repeat 12 months (and yearly)
History and examination	X				
Follow-up assessment		X	X	X	X
Weight/BMI	X	X	X	X	X
Immunocompatibility					
ABO	X				
Repeat ABO	X				
HLA tissue typing	Only at transplant				
PRA and flow cytometry	X				
• >10%	Every 1–2 months				
• VAD	Every 1–2 months				
• Transfusion	2 weeks after transfusion and then 6 months				
Assessment of heart failure severity					
Cardiopulmonary exercise test with RER	X				X
Echocardiogram	X				X
Right heart catheter (vasodilator challenge as indicated)	X		X		X
ECG	X				X
Evaluation of multi-organ function					
Routine lab work	X	X	X	X	X
PT/INR More frequent per protocol if on VAD or coumadin/warfarin	X	X	X	X	X
Urinalysis	X	X	X	X	X
GFR (MDRD equation)	X	X	X	X	X
Unlimed urine sample for protein excretion	X	X	X	X	X
PFT with arterial blood gases	X				
CXR (PA and lateral)	X				
Abdominal ultrasound	X				
Carotid Doppler (if indicated or >50 years)	X				

Table 9.1 (*Contd.*)

Test	Baseline	Repeat			
		3 months	6 months	9 months	12 months (and yearly)
Ankle-brachial index (if indicated or >50 years)	X				
DEXA scan (if indicated or >50 years)	X				
Dental examination	X				X
Ophthalmologic examination (if diabetic)	X				X
Infectious serology and vaccination including:					
Hep B surface Ag	X				
Hep B surface Ab	X				
Hep B core Ab	X				
Hep C Ab	X				
HIV	X				
Syphilis	X				
HSV IgG	X				
CMV IgG	X				
Toxoplasmosis IgG	X				
EBV IgG	X				
Varicella IgG	X				
Tb screen	X				
Influenza vaccine (q 1 year)	X				
Pneumovax (q 5 years)	X				
Hep B immunizations: 1_2_3_	X				
Hep B surface Ab (immunity)	6 weeks after third immunization				
Preventive and malignancy					
Stool for occult blood x 3	X				X
Colonoscopy (if indicated or >50 years)	X				
Mammography (if indicated or >40 years)	X				X
Cervical smear (female ≥18years sexually active)	X				X
PSA and digital rectal exam (men >50 years)	X				X

Reproduced from Mehra MR *et al*. Listing criteria for heart transplantation: International Society for Heart and Lung Transplantation guidelines for the care of cardiac transplant candidates—2006. *J Heart Lung Transplant* 2006; 25: 1024–42 with permission from Elsevier.

Donor compatibility

- Principal match is ABO blood group.
- Other important factors include size-matching for height and weight (±20% and 10%, respectively).
- HLA matching is only performed if panel-reactive antibody >10%.

The CTx procedure

98% of CTx are orthotopic (recipient heart is replaced by donor heart).
- Immediate pre-transplant blood tests:
  - Full blood count, U&Es, LFTs.
  - Coagulation screen.
  - Crossmatch for 4 units (CMV appropriate).
  - Check virology screen.
- Prior to the procedure, the immunosuppressive regime is commenced and antibiotics given according to local protocol, for example,
  - Cefuroxime 1.5g IM/IV as soon as possible.
  - Azathioprine 2mg/kg at induction of anaesthesia.
  - Methylprednisolone 1g at release of aortic cross clamp.

Immediate post-transplant management

- Prophylactic antibiotics, for example, cefuroxime 750mg tds IV for 48 hours, or as long as central venous lines are *in situ*.
- Careful fluid and electrolyte balance must be observed.
- Sliding-scale insulin infusion to maintain tight glycaemic control, will be required for most patients who receive the initially high dose of steroids.
- Continue immunosuppressive regime according to local protocol.

Key reference
Mosteller RD. Simplified calculation of body-surface area. *N Engl J Med* 1987; **317**: 1098.

Commonly used immunosuppressive agents

Corticosteroids

- Intra-operative: 1g methylprednisolone at release of crossclamp.
- Days 1 and 2: 125mg methylprednisolone IV 12-hourly, then oral prednisolone 60mg/day decreasing by 5mg each day and then stopped.
- Thereafter, steroids given for acute rejection (given IV).

Azathioprine

- Antiproliferative immunosuppressant.
- Day 0: 4mg/kg IV at induction.
- Post-operatively: 2mg/kg/day as a single dose if white cell count >4.
- Discontinued when mycophenolate mofetil commenced.
- ► TPMT deficiency suggests risk of azathioprine toxicity.

Mycophenolate mofetil (MMF)

- Antiproliferative immunosuppressant.
- As soon as the patient is able to take oral medications, MMF is commenced at a dose of 1.5g bd (within 5 days of transplant).

Cyclosporin (ciclosporin) A

- Calcineurin inhibitor.
- Commenced when haemodynamics are stable, without evidence of hepatic or renal failure.
- Starting dose: 4mg/kg/day orally or 1.5mg/kg/day IV in two divided doses (the IV dose is approximately a third of the oral dose).
- Subsequent dose depends on blood levels and renal function, and can be measured in two ways:
  - C_0—trough level.
  - C_2—2 hours post dose.
- Target C_0 levels:
  - 300–400µg/L for the first 4 weeks.
  - 200–250µg/L from 4 weeks to 6 months.
  - 150–200µg/L from 6 months to 1 year.
  - 100–150µg/L after 1 year.

Tacrolimus

- Calcineurin inhibitor.
- Alternative to cyclosporin.
- 0.15–0.3mg/kg/day orally as two divided doses.

Endomyocardial biopsy (📖 see Chapter 27)

Patients undergo endomyocardial biopsy to assess for cellular rejection as per local protocol, for example:
- Weekly, for the first 6 weeks.
- Fortnightly, from 6 weeks to 3 months.
- Six-weekly, up to 1 year.
- Thereafter, only when rejection is clinically suspected.

Post-transplant complications

Cardiac transplantation is not without risk—both in the short and long term. There are many post-operative complications, the majority of which are due to immunosuppressive therapy (Table 9.2).

Table 9.2 Post-transplant complications

Complication	Cause
Acute rejection	Host's immune response to donor heart
Infection	Immunosuppression leads to increased risk of infection, including opportunistic infections, for example, CMV, PCP, and toxoplasma
Hypertension	This occurs in 50–90% of all transplant recipients due to cyclosporin therapy, as well as steroids
Renal dysfunction	Due to decreased renal perfusion in heart failure, this often predates transplantation but is exacerbated by cardiopulmonary bypass and cyclosporin therapy
Graft vasculopathy	Accelerated coronary disease, possibly as a result of chronic rejection
Malignancy	Long-term immunosuppression predisposes to a higher risk of neoplasia, particularly cutaneous malignancy and lymphoma
Osteoporosis	Steroid use following CTx, as well as immobility with CHF
Hyperlipidaemia	Steroid therapy often causes a rise in lipid levels
Gout	Cyclosporin causes hyperuricaemia

Management of acute rejection

Clinical signs suspicious of rejection include:
- Pyrexia.
- Atrial arrhythmias.
- Changes in ECG voltage.
- Third heart sound.
- Heart failure.

Grades of cellular rejection on endomyocardial biopsy (ISHLT scale):
- **0**—no rejection.
- **Ia**—focal infiltrate without necrosis.
- **Ib**—diffuse but sparse infiltrate but without necrosis.
- **II**—one focus only, with aggressive infiltration and/or focal myocyte damage.
- **IIIa**—multifocal aggressive infiltrates and/or myocyte damage.
- **IIIb**—diffuse inflammatory process with necrosis.
- **IV**—diffuse aggressive polymorphous infiltrate, and/or oedema, and/or haemorrhage, and/or vasculitis, with necrosis.

Local policy varies as to which grade of rejection should be accepted as indicative of acute rejection, but specific therapy is certainly indicated with biopsy grade ≥IIIa.

Treatment:
- Maintain oral immunosuppressive therapy at optimum levels.
- One of the following additional measures is prescribed:
  - Corticosteroids—methylprednisolone 1g IV daily for 3 days.
  - Antithymocyte globulin (ATG) 0.5mL/kg/day for 3 days.
  - OKT3 monoclonal antibody.
  - Total lymphoid irradiation.
  - Tacrolimus.

Section II

Chronic heart failure and co-morbid conditions

The patient with CHF and angina

Introduction

The most common cause of CHF in westernized countries is ischaemic cardiomyopathy. Many of these patients have had previous myocardial infarction and are no longer troubled by anginal symptoms. As discussed in Chapter 1, the rigour with which the diagnosis of IHD is sought varies from centre to centre. Some perform diagnostic coronary angiography in all HF subjects whereas others restrict the procedure to those with chest pain or evidence of ischaemia on non-invasive testing (exercise testing or myocardial perfusion imaging). The latter approach is often applied in those with comorbidities which may increase the complication rate of angiography.

However, it is important to recognize that all patients, irrespective of the primary aetiology of the CHF, may at some point develop angina due to coronary disease. Untreated, this could progress to cause further myocardial damage with deterioration of the heart failure.

If a patient with CHF attends the clinic and reports having chest pain, the initial steps should be towards establishing whether this pain is cardiac in origin and then deciding how best to manage it.

Investigation

The initial investigation of the patient with CHF and chest pain is similar to that of the patient without CHF:

- History including risk factors:
  - Smoking.
  - Hyperlipidaemia.
  - Diabetes mellitus.
  - Hypertension.
  - Obesity.
  - Physical inactivity.
- Examination.
- Haematology and biochemistry profile.
- ECG.
- Echo.
- Exercise-tolerance test with or without myocardial perfusion imaging.

Further investigation depends on the results. If a non-cardiac cause of chest pain is suspected, for example, oesophageal pain, then further steps should be directed towards establishing that diagnosis.

Chest pain that is thought to be cardiac in origin should, based on international guidelines, suggest that coronary angiography be performed.

Management

The key difference in the management of a patient with CHF and angina from that of a patient without angina is that fluid management is important in optimizing their anginal symptoms. The reductions in ventricular size and pressures associated with achieving euvolaemia have an anti-anginal effect in themselves.

Risk factors for coronary artery disease should be identified and aggressively treated.

Non-pharmacological options
- Weight loss:
  - Obese patients—aim to achieve a target within 10% of ideal body weight.
- Smoking cessation.
- Increase in exercise.

Pharmacological options
At present, all patients should receive all of the following, unless there are specific contra-indications:
- Anti-platelet therapy: aspirin and/or clopidogrel.
- Statin.
- β-Adrenoreceptor antagonist: preferably bisoprolol.
- ACE inhibitor.

In addition, if the symptoms of angina remain poorly controlled, then a long-acting **nitrate** can be added to therapy. This does not confer any survival benefit but has been demonstrated to be tolerated and improve symptoms in patients with angina and reduced LVEF.

Nicorandil has evidence of survival benefit in the management of chronic stable angina. There is no randomized trial evidence of its use in patients with angina and CHF. Care should be taken, if using nicorandil in these patients, due to the blood pressure-lowering side-effect.

In β-adrenoreceptor antagonist-intolerant patients, most calcium channel blockers should be used with caution because of their negative inotropic effect. **Amlodipine** and felodipine can be used in patients with angina and CHF in whom β-blockers and nitrates have not been tolerated.

There has been concern that **aspirin** may attenuate the beneficial effects of ACE inhibitors. Despite these concerns, current guidelines advocate the use of aspirin (75–81mg) in all patients with coronary artery disease and CHF. In aspirin-intolerant patients **clopidogrel** is an acceptable substitute. There is an evidence for dual anti-platelet cover in the acute coronary syndrome population and local guidelines should be considered. Warfarin is an alternative for those intolerant of both of these agents.

Statins are controversial at present in the CHF population. Epidemiological studies have demonstrated an association between low cholesterol and poor prognosis. There have also been suggestions that statins are associated with reduced endotoxin removal, which may be important in patients with gastrointestinal oedema with potential for bacterial translocation. Also, statins reduce levels of ubiquinone and coenzyme Q, and this has been associated with reduced muscle function of both myocardium and skeletal muscle. Two trials are awaited to clarify the place of statins in CHF—CORONA and GISSI-HF.

Interventional options

Patients with angina and CHF whose angiogram demonstrates targets for revascularization should be considered for intervention if they have

- Refractory angina
- Acute coronary syndrome or
- Evidence of viable myocardium (see Chapter 8).

The optimal method of revascularization (CABG or PCI) is the subject of two ongoing international trials: STICH and HEART-UK. CABG has been shown to reduce the risk of death and improve angina symptoms in patients with multi-vessel disease.

Chapter 11

The patient with CHF and arrhythmias

Introduction

Chronic heart failure and arrhythmias often coexist. These include brady-arrhythmias and tachyarrhythmias of both ventricular and supraventricular origin. Up to 50% of deaths in the heart failure population are sudden and unexpected. Sudden cardiac death is between six and nine times more common than in the general population.

Heart failure predisposes patients to arrhythmias; however, arrhythmias also predispose them to heart failure. There are pathological processes that may be common to both diseases, including

- Myocardial fibrosis.
- Alterations in intracellular calcium handling with changes in the action potential.
- Alterations in neuroendocrine function.
- Alterations in sympathetic tone.

Furthermore, the treatment of both bradyarrhythmias and tachyarrhythmias may result in deterioration of left-ventricular systolic function, that in itself is proarrhythmic.

The multifactorial nature of arrhythmias in heart failure has resulted in the 'multi-hit' hypothesis illustrated in Fig. 11.1 which was originally developed to describe the occurrence of sudden cardiac death but which could, as easily, pertain to the relation of arrhythmias in heart failure.

The assessment and management of arrhythmias should be integral to heart-failure care. This includes prevention, accurate diagnosis, and intervention, both pharmacological and device-based.

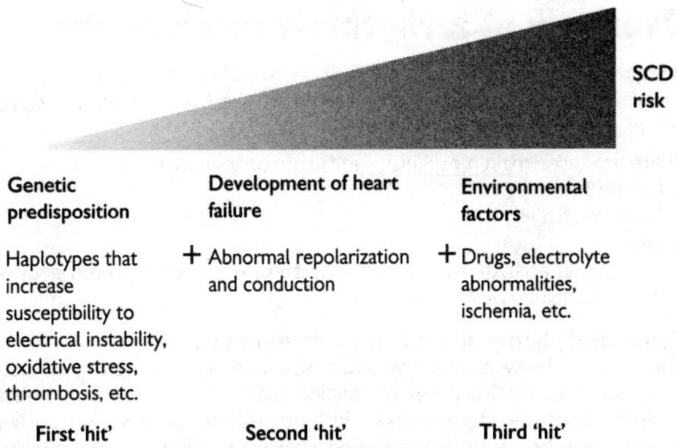

Fig. 11.1 Multi-hit hypothesis of the development of SCD. Heart failure serves to enhance the risk by the associated alterations in the myocardial substrate and increasing the frequency/intensity of triggers of malignant arrhythmias. Reproduced from Tomaselli GF & Zipes DP. What causes sudden cardiac death in heart failure? *Circ Res* 2004; **95**: 754–63 with permission from Lippincott, Williams and Wilkins.

Overview of arrhythmia mechanisms

Arrhythmias are common in CHF irrespective of the aetiology. Although there are multiple factors that contribute to the pro-arrhythmic state, not all of these factors are modifiable.

There are three main mechanisms for ventricular arrhythmias:
- Automatism.
- Triggered activity.
- Re-entry.

In general, an arrhythmia is initiated by automatism or triggered activity and then sustained by re-entry.

Structural change in ischaemic cardiomyopathy

The interface between the myocardial scar and non-infarcted tissue acts as a source of unidirectional conduction block, slow conduction, and a heterogeneous refractory period, with potential for re-entry. This border zone can also be a source of triggered activity, providing an extra stimulus that initiates re-entry to sustain an arrhythmia. Non-infarcted tissue also remodels with gradual hypertrophy of the non-infarcted ventricular cardiomyocytes as they adapt to the increased workload. This hypertrophy in itself may be pro-arrhythmic.

Structural change in non-ischaemic cardiomyopathy

There are extensive changes in the myocardial structure that result in a substrate for re-entry, including fibrosis and altered cell-to-cell coupling, with changes in the expression of connexins 43 and 45.

Automatism is apparent in the sino-atrial node as the pacemaker function. This is determined by the expression of channel proteins, including deactivation of the delayed K^+ current (I_{Kr} or I_{Ks}), activation of the pacemaker current, I_f, and activation of the T-type calcium channel, I_{CaT}.

Under normal conditions, automatism is inhibited in ventricular cells by high K^+ conductance, which keeps the membrane hyperpolarized. The pacemaker current, I_f, is absent or its activation voltage is too negative. However, in pathological conditions such as ischaemic cardiomyopathy, it may be reexpressed or its activation potential may be less negative.

There are two types of triggered activity: early after-depolarizations (EADs) and delayed after-depolarizations (DADs). The main mechanism in EADs is reactivation of the calcium current. These can also be induced by acceleration of the stimulation rate, especially when the cell is in a state of calcium overload. EADs that are independent of $[Ca^{2+}]_i$ can occur especially in heart failure.

DADs are triggered by spontaneous release of Ca^{2+} from the sarcoplasmic reticulum in conditions of Ca^{2+} overload. Ventricular DADs are primarily due to $I_{Na/Ca}$. In heart failure, the Na/Ca exchanger is up-regulated and I_{K1} (the inward rectifier current) is decreased. This destabilizes the membrane potential and results in increased triggered arrhythmias in heart failure.

It has been postulated that triggered activity is responsible for the initiation of almost all arrhythmias in non-ischaemic heart failure and about 50% of those in ischaemic heart failure.

Bradyarrhythmias

The incidence of bradyarrhythmias associated with heart failure is increasing, reflecting the escalating use of β-adrenoreceptor antagonists. Profound bradycardias may result in clinical heart failure, as may be seen in the context of complete heart block.

Heart failure may result from the management of bradycardia. In 1925, Wiggers demonstrated that external stimulation of ventricular myocardium results in adverse changes in haemodynamics. These results have been replicated in several studies and, most recently, this was shown in the DAVID trial which was terminated prematurely.

This trial compared VVI pacing (lower rate limit of 40bpm) with DDDR pacing (lower rate limit of 70bpm) after implantation of an ICD. At the time of data analysis, it was realized that the DDDR group had been paced 60% of the time, while the VVI group was only paced 1% of the time. This has meant that the study is considered to demonstrate the effect of DDDR pacing compared with sinus rhythm. A significantly higher number of patients died or were hospitalized with heart failure in the group of people who were DDDR paced (27% versus 16% in the VVI group). Such pacing is thought to induce mechanical dyssynchrony by effectively causing LBBB. Therefore, standard dual-chamber pacing is not recommended as a therapy for heart failure.

The use of pacemakers to facilitate more aggressive β-adrenoreceptor blockade is not advised. Therefore, the target is to escalate the dose to the maximum-tolerated level based on heart rate, blood pressure, and symptoms.

In patients who require pacing for the treatment of bradycardia, consideration should be made as to whether they qualify for CRT. If not, then dual chamber pacing should be used as backup only with pacing algorithms set to minimize paced beats. Trials are currently underway to compare CRT with DDDR pacing for bradycardia pacing in heart failure patients.

Key references

Sweeney MO & Prinzen FW. A new paradigm for physiologic ventricular pacing. *J Am Coll Cardiol* 2006; **47**: 282–8.

Wilkoff BL, Cook JR, Epstein AE *et al.* Dual-chamber pacing or ventricular backup pacing in patients with an implantable defibrillator: the Dual Chamber and VVI Implantable Defibrillator (DAVID) Trial. *JAMA* 2002; **288**: 3115–23.

Tachycardias

Tachycardias may cause heart failure, as described by tachycardia-induced heart failure or tachycardiomyopathy. Tachycardias are also frequently associated with heart failure. The management of the arrhythmia may directly impact on systolic function, and many anti-arrhythmics are negatively inotropic. Finally, heart failure may result in tachycardias including both atrial and ventricular fibrillation.

Supraventricular tachyarrhythmias

Tachycardiomyopathy most frequently results from incessant atrial arrhythmias. The importance of the diagnosis lies in the recognition that it may be curable by radiofrequency ablation and that ventricular function may return to normal. Frequently, the diagnosis is suspected when the LV systolic dysfunction is noted in combination with persistent tachycardia. The treatment initially centres on standard management of heart failure and negative chronotropic medication. The use of β-adrenoreceptor blockers often achieves both these goals. The exact nature of the arrhythmia will determine the optimal definitive treatment strategy, but this should be planned with an electrophysiologist.

One of the most common supraventricular arrhythmias associated with heart failure is atrial fibrillation that will be discussed on (📖 p. 156). Other supraventricular arrhythmias include atrial flutter and atrial tachycardias. The management of these arrhythmias focuses on restoration of sinus rhythm and prevention of recurrence of arrhythmia. Because of negative inotropic effects, calcium channel blockers should be avoided. The use of class I anti-arrhythmics is similarly discouraged. Therefore, the most useful agents are amiodarone and β-adrenoreceptor blockers. Digoxin may be used to achieve rate-control but does not facilitate cardioversion or maintenance of sinus rhythm. Electrical cardioversion may be used to achieve sinus rhythm.

The role of anticoagulation in atrial flutter and atrial tachycarclia is less clear than in atrial fibrillation. The presence of left ventricular systolic dysfunction is generally accepted as an indication that the risk of thromboembolism is significant. These patients should have consideration of anticoagulation irrespective of planned electrical cardioversion.

Key references

Silverman DI & Manning WJ. Prophylactic anticoagulation of atrial flutter prior to cardioversion: meeting the "burden of proof". *Am J Med* 2001; **111**: 493–4.

Umano E, Solares CA & Alpert MA. Tachycardia-induced cardiomyopathy. *Am J Med* 2003; **114**: 51–5.

Atrial fibrillation and CHF

Atrial fibrillation (AF) and heart failure frequently coexist. They each predispose to the other. The prevalence of AF in LV systolic dysfunction is between 4 and 50%, becoming increasing common in more advanced heart failure. AF is also associated with CHF and preserved LV systolic function. Recent studies have not shown AF to be an independent predictor of increased mortality in patients with CHF.

AF has multiple mechanisms that contribute to heart failure, including the following:

- Loss of atrial contraction that contributes up to 20% of optimal ventricular filling.
- An irregular ventricular rhythm.
- Tachycardia.
- Activation of neurohumoral systems.

Both ACE inhibitors and angiotensin receptor blockers have been shown to reduce the likelihood of developing AF, and this reiterates the importance of these agents in the management of CHF.

There has been extensive discussion about the optimal management strategy for patients with AF, debating rate control and rhythm control. The two key trials in recent years that have considered these questions are RACE and AFFIRM. In the study population as a whole, no significant difference was seen between the two strategies. The difficulty with both these trials is that there was a difference in the anticoagulation strategy between the rate control and the rhythm control arms, this then impacted on the endpoints in the arms as there was an increase in embolic events in the rhythm control limb where the anticoagulation was not continued (Fig. 11.2).

Significant concerns have been raised that the results of these two trials cannot be extrapolated to the CHF population. There is concern that the CHF patients should be treated more aggressively with a goal of restoring and maintaining sinus rhythm in order to improve LV systolic function. Reanalysis of the 26% of patients in the AFFIRM study who had LV systolic dysfunction is underway, and there is a specific trial that will consider the optimal management of AF in patients with NYHA II–IV heart failure and an LVEF <35% (AF-CHF trial).

Rate control can usually be achieved with β-adrenoreceptor blockers ± digoxin. Studies have demonstrated that atrioventricular nodal ablation for the management of AF followed by RV apical pacing is associated with deterioration in heart failure symptoms and LV systolic function. An alternative strategy is ablation of the atrioventricular node followed by cardiac resynchronization therapy. This strategy is currently being studied in the AVERT-AF trial.

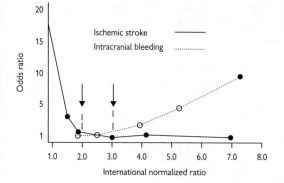

Fig. 11.2 Adjusted odds ratios for ischemic stroke and intracranial bleeding in relation to intensity of anticoagulation. Reproduced from Fuster V *et al.* ACC/AHA/ESC 2006 guidelines for the management of patients with atrial fibrillation—executive summary: a report of the American College of Cardiology/ American Heart Association Task Force on Practice Guidelines and the European Society of Cardiology Committee for Practice Guidelines (Writing Committee to Revise the 2001 Guidelines for the Management of Patients With Atrial Fibrillation). *J Am Coll Cardiol* 2006; **48**: 854–906 with permission from Elsevier.

Key references

Healey JS *et al.* Prevention of atrial fibrillation with angiotensin-converting enzyme inhibitors and angiotensin receptor blockers: a meta-analysis. *J Am Coll Cardiol* 2005; **45**: 1832–9.

Nattel S & Opie LH. Controversies in atrial fibrillation. *Lancet* 2006; **367**: 262–72.

Tops LF *et al.* Right ventricular pacing can induce ventricular dyssynchrony in patients with atrial fibrillation after atrioventricular node ablation. *J Am Coll Cardiol* 2006; **48**: 1642–8.

Van Gelder IC *et al.* A comparison of rate control and rhythm control in patients with recurrent persistent atrial fibrillation (RACE). *N Engl J Med* 2002; **347**: 1834–40.

Wyse DG *et al.* A comparison of rate control and rhythm control in patients with atrial fibrillation. *N Engl J Med* 2002; **347**: 1825–33.

Rhythm control in CHF can be attempted using pharmacology, electrical cardioversion, or radiofrequency ablation. There are ongoing trials to assess the role of pulmonary vein isolation in the treatment of AF in patients with CHF.

Pharmacological options recommended by the ACC/AHA/ESC guidelines (Fig. 11.3) include amiodarone and dofetilide. Amiodarone is safe in patients with heart failure as it has little pro-arrhythmic effect. It does, however, have considerable non-cardiac side-effects. These include corneal deposits, thyroid disease, pulmonary fibrosis, hepatitis and cirrhosis, neuropathy, and photosensitivity. The interaction of amiodarone and warfarin is important as there is an increased anticoagulant effect. Close monitoring of the INR during the initiation of amiodarone is essential. Dofetilide is a class III anti-arrhythmic that blocks the delayed rectifier cardiac potassium channel and prolongs repolarization. It is not currently licensed for use in the UK. Sotalol is no longer considered as a first-line option due to potential pro-arrhythmic effects.

Pharmacological cardioversion of AF is most effective when it occurs within the acute setting. In the context of the patient with CHF, attempted cardioversion AF of less than 48 hours duration can be performed with intravenous or oral amiodarone; however, the patient should then receive anticoagulation to cover the potential recurrence of AF.

Electrical cardioversion of AF may be considered acutely in patients with evidence of shock attributable to the onset of AF with fast ventricular heart rate. More commonly, it is used in persistent AF after a period of anticoagulation to reduce the risk of thromboembolism. Studies have shown that initial synchronized shock energy of 200J for monophasic defibrillators and 100J for biphasic defibrillators has been shown to be associated with an improved success with reduced total shock energy.

Anticoagulation remains an important issue in the care of AF and CHF, whether the AF is paroxysmal, persistent, or permanent. The combination of AF and CHF suggests a significant risk of thromboembolism, such that formal anticoagulation is advised (Fig. 11.2). This is usually achieved with warfarin at a target INR of 2.5. Following cardioversion to sinus rhythm, the anticoagulation should be continued. At present, the duration of therapy is not clear, with some suggesting that the frequency of recurrence of AF in patients with CHF should support the use of warfarin, long-term.

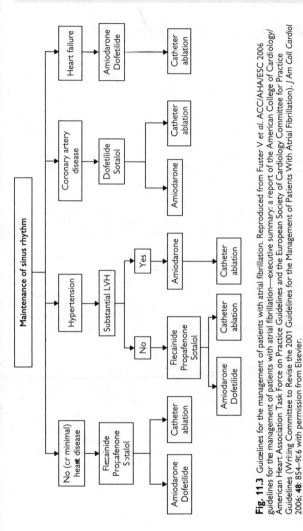

Fig. 11.3 Guidelines for the management of patients with atrial fibrillation. Reproduced from Fuster V et al. ACC/AHA/ESC 2006 guidelines for the management of patients with atrial fibrillation—executive summary: a report of the American College of Cardiology/American Heart Association Task Force on Practice Guidelines and the European Society of Cardiology Committee for Practice Guidelines (Writing Committee to Revise the 2001 Guidelines for the Management of Patients With Atrial Fibrillation). *J Am Coll Cardiol* 2006; **48**: 854–906 with permission from Elsevier.

Key reference

Torp-Pedersen C et al. Dofetilide in patients with congestive heart failure and left ventricular dysfunction. Danish Investigations of Arrhythmia and Mortality on Dofetilide Study Group. *N Engl J Med* 1999; 341: 857–65.

Ventricular tachyarrhythmias

The association of ventricular tachyarrhythmias and heart failure is well established (Fig. 11.4). At least 50% of deaths in the CHF population are thought to be sudden cardiac death, most often ventricular tachyarrhythmias.

Ventricular tachycardia can cause a tachycardiomyopathy if it is incessant or there are frequent paroxysms. In fact, there is evidence that tachycardiomyopathy may even result from frequent ventricular ectopics. The focus of the ventricular tachycardia that is stable enough to induce tachycardiomyopathy is most often from the right-ventricular outflow tract and has a specific morphology: LBBB with an inferior axis. This is an important finding as it can be cured with radiofrequency ablation and the LV systolic function is likely to return to normal.

With the exception of ACE inhibitors, aldosterone antagonists, and β-adrenoreceptor blockers, pharmacological agents have not been shown to improve outcome in the management of ventricular arrhythmias. In fact, many antiarrhythmic agents increase the likelihood of sudden cardiac death because of their pro-arrhythmic effect.

The SCD-HeFT trial has simplified the management of ventricular arrhythmias in patients with an LVEF ≤35%. This study looked at both ischaemic **and** non-ischaemic cardiomyopathies and demonstrated that in those patients with NYHA II or III symptoms there was an absolute risk reduction in mortality at 5 years of 7.2% (29% in the ICD arm versus 36% in the placebo arm). The MADIT and MUSTT trials were studies of ICDs, post-myocardial infarction rather than in CHF; however, they confirm that there is mortality benefit in treating patients with an LVEF ≤30%.

In patients with CHF on optimal medical therapy with QRS duration ≥150ms (or ≥120ms with evidence of ventricular dyssynchrony), the CARE-HF arm demonstrated mortality benefit with CRT-P. The COMPANION study suggested that CRT-D reduced mortality in patients with NYHA III–IV CHF, QRS duration ≥120ms and LVEF ≤35%.

Amiodarone or β-adrenoreceptor blockers can be used in combination with device therapy (ICD or CRT-D) to reduce the frequency of patient events; however, SCD-HeFT demonstrated that amiodarone does not confer additional mortality benefit over best medical therapy (Fig. 11.5).

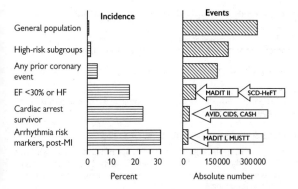

Fig. 11.4 Absolute numbers of arrhythmic events in different patient groups. Reproduced from ACC/AHA/ESC 2006 guidelines for management of patients with ventricular arrhythmias and the prevention of sudden cardiac death. *J Am Coll Cardiol* 2006; **48**: 854–906 with permission from Elsevier.

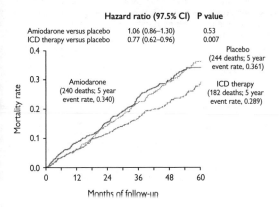

Fig.11.5 Kaplan–Meier graph of death from any cause in the SCD-HeFT trial. Reproduced from Bardy GH et al. Amiodarone or an implantable cardioverter-defibrillator for congestive heart failure. *N Engl J Med* 2005; **352**: 225–37 with permission from Massacheussets Medical Society.

NICE guideline for implantation of ICD in ischaemic CHF

2° prevention
- Survivors of VT/VF cardiac arrest.
- Spontaneous sustained VT with syncope or haemodynamic compromise.
- Sustained VT and LVEF <35% and NYHA <IV.

1° prevention
- LVEF <35% (NYHA <IV) + NSVT on Holter monitor + inducible VT at electrophysiology study.

or

- LVEF <30% (NYHA <IV) + QRS duration ≥120ms.

There is no current NICE guidance for the use of ICDs in non-ischaemic CHF. Based on the results of the SCD-HeFT study, ICDs have a proven mortality benefit in the 1° prevention of ventricular arrhythmias in patients with all of the following:
- Non-ischaemic cardiomyopathy.
- NYHA class II–III.
- LVEF ≤35%.

The cost implications of widespread use of ICDs or CRT-D have driven the search for a means of identifying those *not* at risk of ventricular arrhythmias who do not need an ICD. Work is in progress, but the most promising indicator at present is microvolt T-wave alternans.

Key reference

Chow T et al. Prognostic utility of microvolt T-wave alternans in risk stratification of patients with ischemic cardiomyopathy. *J Am Coll Cardiol* 2006; **47**: 1820–7.

The patient with CHF and arthritis

Introduction

Arthritis can take many forms. Osteoarthritis is a frequent accompaniment to the ageing process. The interaction between inflammatory arthritis and heart failure is multi-faceted, and continues to unfold at both pre-clinical and clinical trial levels:

- Chronic low-grade inflammation is associated with heart failure.
- Chronic low-grade inflammation is associated with atherosclerosis.
- Some treatments can be detrimental to fluid balance.
- Some of the treatments can cause an increase in cardiovascular events.

The balance between what is best in terms of cardiovascular status and maintenance of mobility can be difficult to achieve. In order to ensure optimal management, the treatment of patients with arthritis and heart failure should be coordinated both by a rheumatologist and cardiologist. Informed discussions with the patient are important in establishing a treatment plan.

Cardiovascular disease and inflammatory arthritides

There is an increasing body of evidence supporting the hypothesis that cytokine-driven inflammation is central in the pathogenesis not only of rheumatoid arthritis (RhA) and systemic lupus erythematosis (SLE), but also atherosclerosis and heart failure. The levels of inflammatory mediators are orders of magnitude greater in the rheumatological conditions compared with the cardiac diseases. Therefore, one can hypothesize the interactions between these conditions. Inflammatory arthritis may initiate or promote cardiovascular disease through prolonged exposure to cytokines and related inflammatory mediators.

Both SLE and RhA (and any of the other inflammatory arthritis conditions) have multiple cardiac manifestations including the following conditions:
- Pericarditis.
- Valvular heart disease (most often affecting the mitral valve).
- Myocarditis.
- Cardiac amyloidosis.
- Arrhythmias.
- Coronary artery vasculitis.
- Ischaemic heart disease.

Ischaemic heart disease and ischaemic cardiomyopathy are more frequent and have an increased mortality in patients with inflammatory joint diseases than the general population. Epidemiological and clinical studies indicate that RhA is an independent risk factor for cardiovascular disease. The literature is not conclusive regarding increased incidence of conventional cardiovascular risk factors (see next section). This again supports the central role of inflammatory mediators. Atorvastatin, ACEI, and ARBs are beneficial in reducing synovitis in RhA and modifying vascular risk factors, and this may offer a combined strategy for these patients.

CVS risk factors in inflammatory arthritis
- Probably, ↑ smoking rates in rheumatoid arthritis.
- ↑ Diastolic BP.
- Inflammation tends to:
  - ↓ Total cholesterol
  - ↓↓ HDL
  - ↑ oxidized LDL.

Overall, there is a pro-atherogenic effect with inflammatory arthritis. There is an increasing body of evidence suggesting that novel CVS risk factors, including endothelial dysfunction and insulin resistance, are more significant in the inflammatory arthritides.

Key references

Giles JT et al. Therapy insight: managing cardiovascular risk in patients with rheumatoid arthritis. *Nature Clin Pract Rheum* 2006; **2**: 320–9.

McCarey DW et al. Trial of atorvastatin in rheumatoid arthritis (TARA): double-blind, randomized placebo controlled trial. *Lancet* 2004; **363**: 2015–21.

McEntegart A et al. Cardiovascular risk factors, including thrombotic variables, in a population with rheumatoid arthritis. *Rheumatology (Oxford)* 2001; **40**: 640–4.

Sattar N et al. Explaining how 'high-grade' systemic inflammation accelerates vascular risk in rheumatoid arthritis. *Circulation* 2003; **108**: 2957–63.

Anti-inflammatory drugs and cardiovascular disease

The management of arthritis centres on the control of pain with restoration of function, and reduction of inflammation slowing disease progression.

The drugs in frequent use, as single agents or in combination, include the following:
- Analgesics.
  - Simple, for example, paracetamol (acetaminophen), tramadol.
- NSAIDs.
  - Non-selective.
  - COX-2 selective.
- Steroids.
- Disease-modifying drugs.
  - Hydroxychloroquine.
  - Sulphasalazine.
  - Methotrexate.
  - Gold.
  - Penicillamine.
  - Leflunomide.
  - Steroid sparing (azathioprine and cyclosporin).
- Anti-cytokine agents.
  - Anti-tumour necrosis factor-α agents (etanercept, adalimumab and infliximab).
  - Interleukin-1 receptor antagonists (anakinra).
  - Anti-B cell therapies (rituximab).

Apart from the simple analgesics, all of these agents can have adverse cardiac effects. These are summarized in Table 12.1. In addition, there is a deleterious interaction between aspirin and non-selective NSAIDs including ibuprofen, such that the beneficial effect of aspirin may be attenuated; however, studies suggest that this can be avoided by ensuring that aspirin is taken more than 8 hours before the NSAID.

There is evidence that some of the therapies for arthritis may, in fact, improve the CVS risk profile. For example, methotrexate reduced cardio-vascular deaths in a study of patients with RA. Anti-tumour necrosis factor-α agents increase mortality in established CHF, but may reduce CVS risk in the general RA population.

Table 12.1 Summary of reported cardiovascular side-effects with rheumatological treatments

	Fluid gain/ oedema	CVS vascular events/ vasculitis	Cardiomyopathy
Non-selective NSAIDs	x	x	
COX-2 inhibitors	x	x	
Steroids	x		x
Hydroxychloroquine			x
Methotrexate		x	
Gold	x		
Penicillamine	x		
Leflunomide	x		
Cyclosporin	x		x
Anti-TNF α agents	x	x	x
Rituximab	x	x	x
Azathioprine	Caution with ACEI—may induce anaemia and severe leukopaenia		
Sulphasalazine	Pericarditis with potential for cardiac tamponade		

Key references

Catella-Lawson F et al. Cyclooxygenase inhibitors and the antiplatelet effects of aspirin. N Engl J Med 2001; **345**: 1809–17.

Choi HK et al. Methotrexate and mortality in patients with rheumatoid arthritis: a prospective study. Lancet 2002; **359**: 1173–7.

Dixon WG et al. Rates of MI and CVA in patients with RA treated with Anti-TNF therapy: results from the British Society for Rheumatology Biologics Register. Abstract 681, American College of Rheumatology, Washington 2006.

COX-2 inhibitors and CVS disease

NSAIDs act by inhibiting cyclo-oxygenase (COX) and therefore blocking conversion of arachidonic acid to prostaglandins, prostacyclin, and thromboxanes. There are two isoforms of COX: COX-1 and COX-2. These isoforms are differentially expressed. COX-1 is involved in gastric protection. The most frequent side-effect of non-selective NSAIDs is dyspepsia. The development of COX-2 selective NSAIDs was hoped to herald an end to the gastrointestinal complications.

Risk factors for gastrointestinal bleeding with NSAIDs:
• Age >65 years.
• Anti-thrombotic use.
  • Aspirin.
  • Clopidogrel.
  • Warfarin.
  • Low-molecular weight heparin.
• Corticosteroid use.
• Previous gastrointestinal bleed or active peptic ulcer disease.

The non-selective NSAIDs, including diclofenac and ibuprofen, have not been subjected to such rigorous study as the newer agents. There are NSAIDs considered to be non-selective but that are relatively more selective for COX-2, such as nabumetone and etodolac.

In a recent meta-analysis of COX-2 and traditional/non-selective NSAIDs, the incidence of serious vascular events was similar. The exception appeared to be naproxen, which was associated with the best CVS risk profile and no increase in vascular events. Unfortunately, trials of COX-2 inhibitors have demonstrated an increased risk of cardiovascular events, and this has led to the withdrawal of several agents (Fig. 12.1).
• Rofecoxib was withdrawn from the market in 2004 after a study of colorectal adenomas demonstrated an increase in cardiovascular events approximately double that of the placebo arm. The number-needed-to-harm was 139.
• The MEDAL programme comprised three RCTs totalling 34 701 patients (24 913 with osteoarthritis and 9787 with rheumatoid arthritis). The primary aim was to compare thrombotic CVS events with long-term use of etoricoxib, selective COX-2, and diclofenac.
  • Similar rates of thrombotic cardiovascular events event rates of 1·24 and 1·30 per 100 patient-years, respectively.
  • CHF and oedema were increased with etoricoxib (Fig. 12.2).

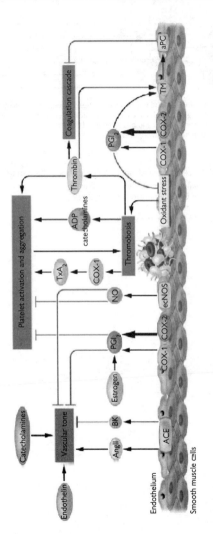

Fig. 12.1 Role of COX-2 in cardiovascular thrombotic events. Reproduced from Grosser T et al. Biological basis for the cardiovascular consequences of COX-2 inhibition: therapeutic challenges and opportunities, J Clin Invest 2006; **116**: 4–15 with permission from Highwire Press.

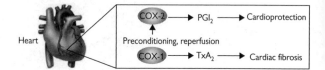

Fig. 12.2 Role of COX-2 in the development of heart failure. Reproduced from Grosser T *et al.* Biological basis for the cardiovascular consequences of COX-2 inhibition: therapeutic challenges and opportunities. *J Clin Invest* 2006; **116**: 4–15 with permission from Highwire Press.

▶▶ All NSAIDs, selective and non-selective, should be avoided when possible in heart failure. They are associated with:
• Deterioration of CHF symptoms with fluid gain.
• Deterioration in renal function.
• Increase in cardiovascular thrombotic events.

Key references

Cannon CP et al. Cardiovascular outcomes with etoricoxib and diclofenac in patients with osteoarthritis and rheumatoid arthritis in the Multinational Etoricoxib and Diclofenac Arthritis Long-term (MEDAL) programme: a randomised comparison. *Lancet* 2006; **368**: 1771–81.

Management of patients with CHF and arthritis

Osteoarthritis

- Simple analgesics should be used, where possible.
- When an NSAID is required, naproxen, even in high dose, is the agent that is not associated with an increase in vascular events. It should, therefore, be used as the first choice NSAID.
- If NSAIDs are required, an assessment of their risk of gastrointestinal bleeding should be made. If they have risk factors for bleeding (see above), then the options are
  - Non-selective NSAIDs + proton-pump inhibitor or H_2 receptor antagonists cover.
  - Non-selective NSAIDs with misoprostol.
  - COX-2 selective NSAIDs.

A recent analysis suggests that the combination of non-selective NSAID and PPI or misoprostol is the most economically appropriate to prevent the need for endoscopy.

Inflammatory arthritis

Management of joint pain should be as above for osteoarthritis.

If there is evidence of pre-existing cardiovascular disease including CHF

- Baseline assessment of cardiovascular status should be performed with:
  - Echo for LVEF.
  - Exercise testing if appropriate and possible.
- COX-2 inhibitors should be avoided.
- Non-selective NSAIDs should be avoided if at all possible, or used at the lowest dose possible for the shortest time. Dosing should be timed to avoid interaction with aspirin (see above).
- Disease-modifying drugs can be used but alterations in diuretic dose may be required.
- Azathioprine should be avoided if concomitant ACE inhibitor is used.
- With the exception of Anakinra, the recombinant human interleukin-1 receptor antagonist, anti-cytokine agents should be avoided if there is evidence of LVSD. If they are to be used then caution is required, and screening echoes performed to assess for deterioration in cardiac status.

If there is no evidence of pre-existing cardiovascular disease

- The development of heart failure symptoms should prompt assessment with echo to confirm the diagnosis.
- Suspicion of drug-induced heart failure should be high and potential agents withdrawn if possible.
- Standard CHF management should be initiated.
- If the patient exhibits symptoms of ischaemic heart disease, coronary angiography is usually appropriate but he or she must be assessed for possible coronary vasculitis.

Gout

Gout is commonly associated with CHF, in part because of elevated plasma urate concentrations secondary to diuretic use. An increased plasma urate concentration has also been associated with an adverse prognosis.

The treatment of gout in the patient with CHF is complicated by the relative contra-indication to NSAIDs, COX-2 inhibitors, and corticosteroids. Therefore, acute exacerbations of gout should be managed with colchicine, and allopurinol is recommended to prevent recurrence.

Colchicine is given as a 1mg initial dose, followed by 500µg every 4 hours to maximum dose of 6mg in 3 days. Patients should be made aware of the common side-effects which include abdominal discomfort, vomiting, and diarrhoea.

Interestingly, several studies have postulated a beneficial effect in CHF of targeted inhibition of xanthine oxidase with allopurinol. The suggested mechanism includes reduction of free radical load and uric acid production; however, this has yet to be substantiated in clinical trials.

Key references

Brown TJ et al. A comparison of the cost-effectiveness of five strategies for the prevention of non-steroidal anti-inflammatory drug-induced gastrointestinal toxicity: a systematic review with economic modeling. *Health Technol Assess* 2006; **10**: 1–202.

Hooper L et al. The effectiveness of five strategies for the prevention of gastrointestinal toxicity induced by non-steroidal anti-inflammatory drugs: systematic review. *BMJ* 2004; **329**: 948.

Kearney PM et al. Do selective cylco-oxygenase-2 inhibitors and traditional non-steroidal anti-inflammatory drugs increase the risk of atherothrombosis? meta-analysis of randomized trials. *BMJ* 2006; **332**: 1302–08.

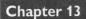

The patient with CHF and anaemia

Introduction

Anaemia is common in patients with chronic heart failure. The proportion of those who have anaemia increases with deteriorating NYHA functional class. A reduced haemoglobin level is also associated with increased symptoms, more frequent hospitalizations and, in most studies, with an increased mortality rate. Severe anaemia can also lead to high-output cardiac failure in the absence of heart disease.

Definition

There is significant variability in the definition of anaemia. The most commonly used definition is that of the WHO, taken from a document on iron deficiency anaemia:

- <12g/dL in women.
- <13g/dL in men.

This definition does not take into account post-menopausal women, a group that some would argue should have a similar haemoglobin to men.

Prevalence

The prevalence of anaemia in heart failure varies considerably between studies, partly due the variability of the definition used; however, on average, around 20% of patients with CHF have anaemia by WHO criteria, the proportion increasing with worsening HF.

Aetiology

The causes of anaemia in CHF are multifactorial, but it is likely that the mechanisms include the following:

- Haemodilution.
- Reduced renal perfusion.
- Reduced bone marrow perfusion.
- Down-regulation of erythropoietin (EPO) by ACE inhibitors.
- Angiotensin receptor blockers.
- Cytokines (e.g. TNF-α).
- ↓ EPO in associated chronic renal disease.
- Iron deficiency caused by aspirin consumption.
- Thalassaemia or other hereditary cause of anaemia.
- Other coexisting haematinic deficiency.

Investigations

- Full blood count.
- Mean corpuscular volume (see next section).
- Haematinics.
- Iron studies.
- Blood film.

Anaemia and mean corpuscular volume (MCV)

Microcytic (low MCV):
- Iron deficiency (by far the commonest cause).
  - Microcytic, hypochromic.
  - Low serum iron.
  - Low ferritin.
  - Raised total iron binding capacity.
- Thalassaemia.
- Congenital sideroblastic anaemia.

Normocytic (normal MCV):
- Anaemia of chronic disease.
- Haemolysis.
- Bone marrow failure.
- Pregnancy.

Macrocytic (high MCV):
- Vitamin B_{12} deficiency.
- Folate deficiency.
- Alcohol excess.
- Hypothyroidism.
- Reticulocytosis (pseudo-macrocytosis).

Key references

Anand IS et al. Anemia and change in hemoglobin over time related to mortality and morbidity in patients with chronic heart failure: results from Val-HeFT. *Circulation* 2005; **112**: 1121–7.

Horwich TB et al. Anemia is associated with worse symptoms, greater impairment in functional capacity and a significant increase in mortality in patients with advanced heart failure. *J Am Coll Cardiol* 2002; **39**: 1780–6.

Prognosis

Many heart failure studies have identified coexisting anaemia as an adverse prognostic sign, with increasing mortality with lower haemoglobins. (see Fig. 13.1).

Treatment

Firstly, treat any reversible causes!

Aim for a haemoglobin >10g/dL, transfusing as appropriate, acknowledging the risks associated with blood products.

There has been significant interest in erythropoietin, given along with iron supplementation, as a possible therapeutic agent in patients with anaemia and CHF. Small non-blinded studies have suggested:
• An improvement in:
  • Hb
  • NYHA class
  • LVEF
  • VO_2.
• A reduction in:
  • Hospitalization
  • Diuretic requirements.

Potential risks of erythropoietin therapy include the following:
• Increased thrombosis (including stroke).
• Platelet activation.
• Hypertension.

▶ Large placebo-controlled, blinded RCTs are needed before EPO is added to the routine armamentarium of heart failure therapy. The RED-HF study comparing s/c darbepoetin-α with placebo in patients with symptomatic LVSD and anaemia began recruitment in 2006. There are also ongoing trials with IV iron.

Suggested dosing of EPO: 60U/kg/week s/c erythropoietin in addition to iron (IV or oral).

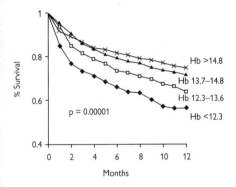

Fig. 13.1 Kaplan–Meier survival analysis in 1061 patients with CHF stratified by Hb quartile. Reproduced from Horwich *et al*. Anemia is associated with worse symptoms, greater impairment in functional capacity and a significant increase in mortality in patients with advanced heart failure. *J Am Coll Cardiol* 2002; **39**: 1780–86 with permission from Elsevier.

Key references

Mancini DM *et al*. Effect of erythropoietin on exercise capacity in patients with moderate to severe chronic heart failure. *Circulation* 2003; **107**: 294–9.

Silverberg DS *et al*. The use of subcutaneous erythropoietin and intravenous iron for the treatment of the anemia of severe, resistant congestive heart failure improves cardiac and renal function and functional cardiac class, and markedly reduces hospitalizations. *J Am Coll Cardiol* 2000; **35**:1737–44.

Silverberg DS *et al*. The effect of correction of mild anemia in severe, resistant congestive heart failure using subcutaneous erythropoietin and intravenous iron: a randomized controlled study. *J Am Coll Cardiol* 2001; **37**: 1775–80.

The patient with CHF and adult congenital heart disease

Introduction

Congenital heart disease has an incidence of approximately 8 cases per 1000 live births. The term congenital heart disease covers a wide spectrum of lesions. At one end are the lesions of such severity that the child dies before reaching adulthood. At the opposite extreme, there are lesions that are small or that spontaneously resolve, for example, small ventricular septal defects. However, the majority of the cases of congenital heart disease require ongoing multidisciplinary input.

The success of surgical and medical management has resulted in over 80% of patients with congenital heart disease reaching the age of 16. There are now more adults with congenital heart disease (i.e. survivors) than there are children.

The growth of the population of adults with congenital heart disease brings new challenges. They require monitoring of their original lesion and the consequences of any surgical repair. The timing and mode of further intervention, either surgical or percutaneous, remains open to debate.

However, it is becoming apparent that the long-term limitation of these patients results from heart failure. The aetiology of the heart failure is different, not the myocardial necrosis of ischaemic cardiomyopathy. The heart failure of adult congenital heart disease (ACHD) results from a lifetime of abnormal cardiac pressure, volume, tension, and flow. The result is a combination of impaired contractility with abnormal preload and afterload.

Studies of heart failure in ACHD are being performed. A recent study examined the aerobic capacity in a range of six lesions:
- Closed atrial septal defect.
- Surgically corrected transposition of the great arteries (Fig. 14.1).
- Congenitally corrected transposition of the great arteries.
- Repaired tetralogy of Fallot (Fig. 14.2).
- Ebstein's anomaly.
- Fontan physiology (univentricular heart with diversion of the systemic venous return to the pulmonary artery).

All six of the groups had a mean peak VO_2 of <22mL/kg/minute, and in the Fontan group the mean peak VO_2 was only 16mL/kg/minute. This is comparable to NYHA III in ischaemic or dilated cardiomyopathy. It has been postulated, because of the fact that such varying anatomical defects can result in reduced aerobic capacity, that the problem lies outside the heart and is related to abnormalities of skeletal muscle—changes that are seen in other heart failure syndromes.

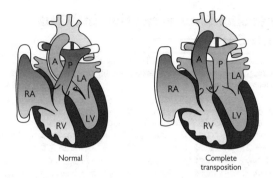

Fig. 14.1 Transposition and a normal heart for comparison. Reproduced from Myerson SG, et al. *Emergencies in Cardiology*, 2005, (📖 p. 229) with permission from Oxford University Press.

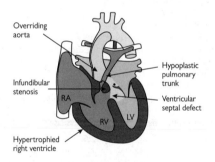

Fig. 14.2 Tetralogy of Fallot. Reproduced from Myerson SG, et al. *Emergencies in Cardiology*, 2005, (📖 p. 233) with permission from Oxford University Press.

Key references

Bolger AP et al. Congenital heart disease: the original heart failure syndrome. *Eur Heart J* 2003; **24**: 970–6.

Fredriksen PM et al. Aerobic capacity in adults with various congenital heart diseases. *Am J Cardiol* 2001; **87**: 310–4.

Neurohumoral activation in ACHD with CHF

'Classical' heart failure is associated with activation of sympathetic nervous system, renin–angiotensin–aldosterone system, endothelin, cytokines and natriuretic peptides.

The role of these pathways in the evolution of heart failure in patients with ACHD has been investigated. Compared to age-matched controls, patients with ACHD had neurohumoral activation increasing in parallel with increasing NYHA class or with deteriorating systemic ventricular function.

In patients with ACHD but without any symptoms of heart failure (NYHA class I) there is evidence of activation of natriuretic peptides, norepinephrine and endothelin-1.

However, while there was neurohumoral activation, there was no difference between four anatomical groups of patients with ACHD:
- Tetralogy of Fallot.
- Systemic right-ventricular physiology.
- Single-ventricular physiology.
- Miscellaneous other lesions.

Neurohumoral activation in patients with ACHD correlated well with other standard measures of heart failure severity including the following:
- Cardiothoracic ratio on CXR.
- QRS duration.
- Right and left atrial volumes.

The combination of neurohumoral activation and reduced aerobic capacity in a patient with ACHD equates with a diagnosis of heart failure, as it would in patients with other forms of cardiac disease.

The nature of the underlying cardiac lesion is important in assessing the likelihood and severity of resultant heart failure. Patients with cyanotic heart disease have lower aerobic capacity and higher neurohormonal activation than acyanotic patients. Patients with Fontan physiology have the most significant limitation in aerobic capacity.

Key references

Bolger AP *et al.* Neurohormonal activation and the chronic heart failure syndrome in adults with congenital heart disease. *Circulation* 2002; **106**: 92–9.

Fredriksen PM *et al.* Aerobic capacity in adults with various congenital heart diseases. *Am J Cardiol* 2001; **87**: 310–4.

Pharmacological options

Standard heart failure therapies have been well proven in the management of the majority of adult heart failure syndromes; however, there is not the same wealth of evidence for their use in patients with CHF as a result of ACHD. These studies are difficult to achieve because of the smaller numbers of patients and the diversity of individual patient's initial presentation and subsequent surgical intervention.

Diuretics These are accepted in the management of symptoms of fluid overload. Loop diuretics are often very effective, although the dose may need to initially be given intravenously if there is chronic peripheral oedema. The main difference in the use of diuretics in this population of patients is that consideration needs to be given to the preload–afterload balance of the individual patient. If they are dependent on their preload for cardiac output then caution must be applied in the prescription of diuretics. The addition of thiazide diuretics should be cautious as hypokalaemia may precipitate life-threatening arrhythmias.

Aldosterone antagonists These have no proven mortality benefit in this population. At higher doses, they may be helpful in the management of patients with severe sub-pulmonic ventricular failure with ascites, or in patients with Fontan physiology who have developed protein-losing enteropathy.

ACE inhibitors and ARBs These are not infrequently used in the patient with CHF and ACHD. There are small studies in patients with specific ACHD lesions that have suggested little benefit in terms of aerobic capacity or haemodynamics; however, these studies were small and mainly retrospective. In systemic right ventricles, there is evidence of benefit with both ACE inhibitors and ARBs. ACE inhibitors improved symptoms and quality of life in a small retrospective study of patients with cyanotic lesions. There is also emerging evidence of benefit in the use of ACE inhibitors in cyanotic patients with nephropathy and proteinuria.

β-blockers There is very little published experience of the use of β-blockers in the management of CHF and ACHD. There is single centre evidence of benefit in their use in patients with left ventricular dysfunction resulting from tetralogy of Fallot and other right-sided congenital heart defects. There is also cautious use in patients with systemic right-ventricular failure, although the dose may be limited by heart block and sinus node dysfunction.

Most specialists caring for patients with ACHD and CHF have taken a pragmatic approach in applying the evidence from the large heart failure trials to their patient group. While one must 'first do no harm', cautious use of these agents tailored to an individual patient appears to be a reasonable strategy. The inclusion of these patients in a registry may establish a body of experience to allow guidelines to be developed.

Assessment of a patient with ACHD and CHF

- Exclude non-cardiac causes for symptoms.
  - Thyroid function.
  - Anaemia.
  - Hypotension.
  - Iatrogenic, for example, side-effects from medication.
- Assess for any haemodynamically significant lesion.
  - Does it require surgery or intervention?
- Is there a dysrhythmia?
  - Does the patient require DC cardioversion?
  - Is there a role for electrophysiology study ± ablation?
- Establish the baseline NYHA status.
  - Consider formal cardiopulmonary exercise testing.
- Introduce tailored pharmacological therapy.
  - ACE inhibitor is often the first drug initiated.
- If there is evidence of dyssynchrony, consider CRT (± D).
- If the condition is deteriorating, consider role of transplantation.
  - Heart/lung/heart-lung?
- Consider end of life issues, including palliative care.

Key references

Book WM. Heart failure in the adult patient with congenital heart disease. *J Cardiac Failure* 2005; **11**: 306–12.

Ringel RE & Peddy SB. Effect of high-dose spironolactone on protein-losing enteropathy in patients with Fontan palliation of complex congenital heart disease. *Am J Cardiol* 2003; **91**: 1031–2.

Interventional options

The development of chronic heart failure in a patient with ACHD requires review by an ACHD specialist. As described previously, the evidence for pharmacological intervention is patchy. Assessment of the patient's anatomy is essential to consider whether further interventions may be beneficial.

Surgical issues In patients with repaired tetralogy of Fallot, the development of pulmonary regurgitation is common. As the regurgitation increases, the RV dilates and fails. Left-ventricular dysfunction has been shown to correlate with RV dysfunction in this group. Pulmonary valve replacement improves right-ventricular function and improves or prevents LVD. It improves aerobic capacity, reduces arrhythmias and prevents further prolongation of the QRS duration. Timing of pulmonary valve replacement can be difficult, but it is optimally performed before irreversible RV dysfunction occurs. Percutaneous pulmonary valve replacements are being used in small numbers of patients.

A systemic morphologic right ventricle is likely to struggle in the long term. As the ventricle dilates it splints the interventricular septum reducing LV size but also inducing LV dysfunction. Pulmonary artery banding was initially intended to 'train' the morphologic LV prior to surgical arterial correction. However it has been recognized that it is a therapeutic intervention in itself. The resistance of the pulmonary outflow forces the LV to remodel and improves its geometry including restoring septal function, which in turn improves the RV (systemic) ventricular function.

In patients who have had baffles or conduits formed (Fig. 14.3) as part of their surgical procedure, CHF can develop gradually due to stenosis. The stenosis may be amenable to percutaneous dilatation ± stenting or may require more complex surgical repair.

Cardiac resynchronization Specific trials of CRT in patients with ACHD have not been performed; however, there is a limited body of experience supporting the use of CRT in ACHD with systemic RV dysfunction. There are also reports of CRT being used in tetralogy of Fallot and also in patients with transposition of the great arteries—either post-Mustard or in complex congenitally corrected TGA. The additional consideration in these patients is how and where to place the leads as the venous anatomy may preclude an entirely endovascular system. Sometimes an epicardial ventricular lead requires to be placed thoracoscopically or via mini-thoracotomy.

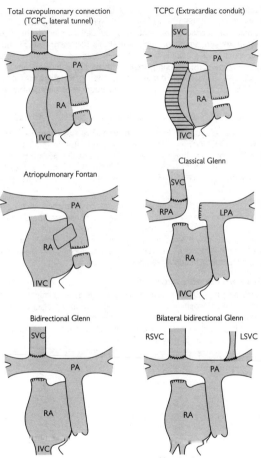

Fig. 14.3 Various Fontan operations. Reproduced from Myerson SG et al. *Emergencies in Cardiology*, 2005, (📖 p. 243) with permission from Oxford University Press.

Key references

Book WM. Heart failure in the adult patient with congenital heart disease. *J Cardiac Failure* 2005; **11**: 306–12.

Dubin AM et al. Electrical resynchronization: a novel therapy for the failing right ventricle. *Circulation* 2003; **107**: 2287–9.

Implantable cardioverter defibrillators. ICDs, with or without cardiac resynchronization, are being considered for patients with ACHD for either primary or secondary prevention of sudden cardiac death. The exact indications and timing of implantation are still being established. The most recent NICE guidelines revised the indications and now suggest that they should be considered in patients with surgical repair of congenital heart disease. It has been demonstrated that in tetralogy of Fallot, QRSd >180ms is associated with an increased risk of ventricular arrhythmia.

The role of atrial ICDs to treat atrial arrhythmias is also being defined.

The role of transplantation. End-stage heart failure can occur in young patients with ACHD. Some of them may be candidates for transplantation in the form of heart, lung, or heart and lung. The decisions regarding transplantation need to be made on an individual patient basis. Early referral to a transplant centre allows consideration of all the issues in a multidisciplinary setting.

The initial diagnosis, surgical interventions, and complications of procedures and therapies can all result in additional problems at the time of transplantation and in the post-operative care. For example, repeated surgical procedures may mean that the patient has limited vascular access, or has had multiple blood and blood product transfusions with resultant hepatitis C infection or multiple preformed antibodies.

Palliative care in end-stage CHF

Care of the patient with end-stage heart failure is as important a stage as the acute care. Recognition that they are in the final stages of their disease and the communication of this is vital to allow the patient and their family time. As discussed in section VII, the involvement of hospice care may be appropriate, as may the use of opiates.

NICE indications for ICDs in ACHD

- 2° prevention
  - Aborted sudden cardiac death
  - Ventricular arrhythmia with syncope
- 1° prevention
  - 'After surgical repair of congenital heart disease'.

Key reference

Lamour JM *et al*. Outcome after orthotopic cardiac transplantation in adults with congenital heart disease. *Circulation* 1999; **100**(Suppl 19): II 200–5.

Pulmonary hypertension in ACHD with CHF

Pulmonary hypertension is defined as an elevation in the *mean* pulmonary artery pressure ≥25mmHg at rest or 30mmHg on exercise.

Pulmonary vascular disease can occur as a consequence of left-to-right flow through an intracardiac shunt, such as a VSD with resultant Eisenmenger's syndrome. It can also occur in association with connective tissue disease or as a primary lesion.

In the context of ACHD, breathlessness may be attributable to ventricular dysfunction or pulmonary hypertension. Both of these conditions may coexist and establishing the relative contributions of each may be challenging. The definition of pulmonary hypertension may be difficult to apply, for example, how does one define pulmonary hypertension in a patient with Fontan physiology?

There are three mechanisms that have been identified as potential therapeutic targets in the management of pulmonary hypertension (Fig. 14.4):
● Endothelin receptors.
● Phosphodiesterase-5.
● Prostacyclins.

Bosentan is an endothelin-1 receptor antagonist that has been shown in the BREATHE-5 study to achieve symptomatic improvement and a significant improvement in pulmonary vascular resistance, pulmonary artery pressure, and 6-minute walk test distance.

Sildenafil is a phosphodiesterase-5 inhibitor that blocks metabolism of nitric oxide. Studies have demonstrated an improvement in aerobic capacity and symptoms.

Prostacyclins are potent vasodilators and inhibitors of platelet activation. They can be given by intravenous infusion, subcutaneous infusion, inhaled aerosol, or oral preparation. Significant improvement has been demonstrated in exercise capacity and cardiopulmonary haemodynamics.

Short-term benefit has been demonstrated with these therapies. Longer follow-up will define the extent of these benefits. Work is ongoing to establish the optimal therapeutic strategy for these patients. Of particular interest is work that considers combinations of these therapies. Many of these patients are anticoagulated if there is any issue regarding pulmonary thromboembolic disease. Indeed, the very dilated pulmonary arteries may form a thrombus in situ. The previous mainstay of therapy, calcium channel blockers are now used for patients with primary pulmonary hypertension who have been demonstrated to have an acute vasodilator response, as assessed with short-acting agents such as inhaled nitric oxide or intravenous prostacyclin at right heart catheterization (Fig. 14.4).

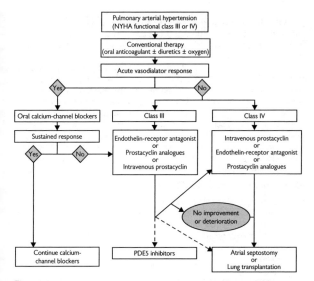

Fig. 14.4 Algorithm for the management of patients with pulmonary hypertension and NYHA class III or IV symptoms. The drugs of choice for testing of acute vasoreactivity are short-acting agents (e.g., intravenous prostacyclin, intravenous adenosine, or inhaled nitric oxide). Patients with a sustained benefit from calcium-channel blockers are defined as those in NYHA functional class I or II who have near-normal hemodynamic values after at least one year of follow-up. Most experts recommend that patients in NYHA functional class IV receive continuous intravenous epoprostenol. Lung transplantation is considered an option for all eligible patients who remain in NYHA IV after three months of receiving epoprostenol. Atrial septostomy is proposed for selected patients with severe disease. Reproduced from Humbert M et al. Treatment of pulmonary arterial hypertension. *N Engl J Med* 2004; **351**: 1425–36.

► **Acute management options of pulmonary hypertension**
- Seek expert help.
- High-flow oxygen
- Consider specific agents: nitric oxide/iloprost/epoprostenol/sildenafil.
- Consider ECMO ± RVAD.
- Consider atrial septostomy.

▶ Acute management of heart failure in ACHD

Although this chapter addresses the patient with CHF and ACHD, it would be inappropriate to overlook the management of the acutely decompensated patient.

⚠ The key issue in the management of these patients is an appreciation of the underlying physiology and then relating this to the acute presentation. Classical signs may be misleading, for example, an elevated JVP is appropriate for a patient with Fontan physiology, and aggressive diuresis to 'treat' it may have disastrous results. Some lesions are likely to result in systemic ventricular failure, presenting with 'left-ventricular failure' signs and symptoms, while others may cause sub-pulmonic ventricular failure, with 'right-heart failure' signs and symptoms. These are summarized below. The most frequent presentation of acute ventricular failure is of sub-pulmonic failure.

▶▶ Early involvement of an ACHD specialist is always appropriate.

The presentation of acute ventricular failure should prompt investigations to identify the cause. The possible causes include:
- Arrhythmias (most common cause).
- Obstruction of conduits.
- Infection.
- Ischaemia.
- Anaemia.
- Pulmonary thromboembolic disease.

ACHD lesions that may cause systemic ventricular failure
- Mitral valve disease.
- Acute severe aortic regurgitation.
- Aortic stenosis.
- Unrepaired coarctation.
- Mustard repair with systemic ventricular failure.
- Congenitally corrected transposition of the great arteries.
- Systemic left-ventricular failure (e.g. elderly Fallot's patient).
- Pulmonary vein obstruction.
- Myocardial disease (e.g. Duchenne muscular dystrophy).

ACHD lesions that may cause sub-pulmonic ventricular failure
- Fontan physiology.
- Pulmonary hypertension.
- Large atrial septal defects.
- Tricuspid valve disease.
- RV-pulmonary artery conduit obstruction (e.g. Rastelli procedure).
- Mustard repair with baffle obstruction.
- Severe pulmonary regurgitation with RV dilatation (e.g. repaired Fallot's).

Reproduced from Gatzoulis MA et al. *Adult Congenital Heart Disease: A Practical Guide*, 2005 with permission from Blackwell Publishing (ISBN 0727916688).

Initial management of the patient presenting in failure centres on initial resuscitation following a standard ABC approach. Thereafter the management needs to be focused on the patient's cardiac lesion. A suggested approach is the following:
• ABC.
• Identify the underlying lesion—what is the anatomy?
  • Does this patient have a Fontan repair?
• Is there an acute haemodynamic lesion that needs urgent intervention (e.g. a ruptured mitral valve chordae)?
• Is the patient in sinus rhythm?
  • This may be difficult to assess, however, even rate-controlled atrial flutter may be detrimental to a patient with Fontan physiology. Obtain a 12-lead ECG to aid diagnosis. If not sinus rhythm, consider urgent cardioversion. Chemical cardioversion is often unsuccessful and so electrical cardioversion should be considered. A TOE may be required to exclude intra-cardiac thrombus first.
• Is there evidence of sepsis—either systemic or endocarditis?
• Where is the problem?
  • Systemic or sub-pulmonic ventricle, or both?
• What is the primary problem?
  • Pulmonary oedema, peripheral oedema, or low cardiac output?

Once all these aspects have been considered specific management can be considered. The role of any drug has to be balanced against potential changes in filling pressures, renal perfusion, etc. Table 14.1 considers the role of various agents in this population of patients.

The final comment is that the venous anatomy of the patient with ACHD is often complex. Femoral veins may have been tied off after cardiac catheterization studies as a child. The head and neck veins may not connect in the expected fashion. Therefore, caution should be applied before placing lines.

▶▶ Early involvement of an ACHD specialist is always appropriate.

Table 14.1 Pharmacological options in HF and ACHD

Drug	Advantages	Disadvantages
Loop diuretics	Effective for symptom control	Caution if pre-load dependent
		Caution if renal dysfunction
		May need IV dosing if chronically oedematous
Spironolactone	Effective for right-sided failure symptom control	
β-blockers	Good for HR control	Caution regarding conduction abnormalities
Digoxin	Rate control for permanent AF	
Nitrates		Rarely used as patients borderline hypotensive
Opiates	May be useful in palliative care of heart failure	

Reproduced from Gatzoulis MA et al. Adult Congenital Heart Disease: A Practical Guide, 2005 with permission from Blackwell Publishing, 2005.

Chapter 15

The patient with CHF and diabetes mellitus

Introduction

Heart failure and diabetes mellitus (DM) commonly coexist, but few clinicians are specialists in both areas. There are difficulties managing these two conditions when they coexist. For example, many of the drugs used to control hyperglycaemia are relatively 'contra-indicated' in HF.

Definition

Diabetes mellitus has been described by the World Health Organization as 'a metabolic disorder of multiple aetiology, characterized by chronic hyperglycaemia with disturbances of carbohydrate, fat and protein metabolism resulting from defects in insulin secretion, insulin action, or both'.

The WHO advises that the range of blood glucose indicative of diabetes mellitus are as follows:

- Random venous plasma glucose ≥11.1mmol/L *or*
- Fasting plasma glucose (FPG) ≥7.0mmol/L *or*
- Plasma glucose ≥11.1mmol/L 2 hours after a 75g oral glucose tolerance test.

Epidemiology

- The prevalence of DM in the general population is approximately 4–7%.
- Approximately 0.3–0.5% of the general population has both HF and DM.
- Around 12% of patients with DM in general population studies have HF, and in patients over 64 years of age, the prevalence of DM in HF rises to 22%.
- The prevalence of DM in populations with LVSD varies from 6 to 25%, increasing in those with symptomatic HF, where the prevalence of DM is between 12 and 30%.
- The risk of developing DM is greatest in more advanced HF.
- 7.4% of patients with HF in the placebo arm of the CHARM programme developed DM over a median follow-up of 3.1 years.

Aetiology

Insulin resistance, impaired fasting glucose, and hyperinsulinaemia in the absence of DM are common in HF. They are also risk factors for HF, independent of DM and other established risk factors.

Insulin resistance occurs in HF of both ischaemic and non-ischaemic aetiology. The relationship is likely to be multifactorial. Possible causes include the following:
- Sympathetic nervous system activation.
- Sedentary lifestyle.
- Endothelial dysfunction.
- Loss of skeletal muscle mass.
- Cytokines (e.g. TNF-α and leptin) on peripheral insulin sensitivity.

Investigations

Investigations indicated in the heart failure patient with diabetes include the following:
- Fasting glucose.
- HbA1c.
- Oral glucose tolerance test.
- Urinalysis.
- Microalbuminuria.
- Fundoscopy.
- Lipids.
- Ferritin.

▶ CHF + DM consider haemachromatosis.

Prognosis

- DM is an independent predictor of mortality in patients with HF.
- HF patients with DM have a consistently higher mortality and HF hospitalization rates than patients without DM.
- Increased mortality seems to be due to death by pump failure only.
- Patients with DM that develop HF have a markedly increased mortality.
- Albuminuria is an independent predictor of first hospitalization for HF in patients with both DM and hypertension, with no previous history of MI or HF.

Management of diabetes in HF

Sulphonylureas

Sulphonylureas stimulate endogenous insulin production. Primarily due to concerns relating to the other classes of oral hypoglycaemic agents, this class of drug is preferentially used in patients with HF.

In a non-randomized cohort study of patients with DM and HF, those with a new diagnosis of HF had a better 1 year mortality on metformin when compared to those on sulphonylureas (adjusted HR 0.66 (0.44–0.97)).

Metformin

The American Diabetic Association guidelines state that metformin is contra-indicated in patients with HF. In the UK, neither the Scottish Intercollegiate Guideline Network nor National Institute for Clinical Excellence, in their DM or HF guidelines, state that metformin is contra-indicated in HF. There are no statements regarding metformin in the ESC or AHA HF guidelines.

Metformin is commonly used in diabetics with heart failure, either alone, or in combination with sulphonylurea or insulin. There is a small risk of lactic acidosis, but this risk does not appear to be high; however, temporary withdrawal during periods of cardiac decompensation may be appropriate.

In retrospective studies, metformin was associated with a reduced mortality and hospitalization in patients with DM and CHF, compared to those treated with sulphonylureas.

Thiazolidinediones (TZDs)

TZDs are peroxisome proliferator-activated (PPAR-γ) receptor agonists. According to a consensus statement published jointly by the ADA/AHA, TZDs can be used cautiously in patients with NYHA class I/II HF, but should not be used in patients with NYHA class III/IV HF due to the fact that TZDs cause an increase in plasma volume, peripheral oedema, and weight gain (averaging between 1 and 3kg). The risk of oedema increases in patients co-administered insulin. Fluid retention was usually quickly reversed upon drug withdrawal and an increase in diuretics.

Insulin

Insulin use has been demonstrated to independently predict both development of HF and mortality in patients with DM; however, it is likely that insulin use is a marker for patients who have DM of longer duration perhaps with more extensive macrovascular disease.

Management of CHF in diabetes

ACE-inhibitors and ARBs

Blocking the RAAS reduces the development of DM in patients with HF. In a retrospective analysis of the SOLVD study, enalapril reduced the incidence of DM when compared to placebo (HR = 0.22 (0.10–0.46), p < 0.0001). In the CHARM study, candesartan also reduced the incidence of DM in patients with HF (HR = 0.78 (0.64–0.96), p = 0.02).

It should also be recognized that ACE inhibitors (micro-HOPE) and ARBs (LIFE), have been shown to reduce the incidence of heart failure in diabetic patients.

β-adrenoreceptor antagonists

Patients with HF and DM are less likely to be discharged from hospital on β-adrenoreceptor antagonists than patients with HF who do not have DM.

The major trials of β-adrenoreceptor antagonists in HF, which demonstrated reductions in mortality and HF hospitalization, included between 12 and 29% of patients with DM, and sub-group analyses suggest that patients with and without DM have similar benefits.

There are concerns that β-adrenoreceptor antagonism may decrease awareness of hypoglycaemia and blunt the compensatory increase in plasma glucose in insulin-treated diabetics; however, this appears to be less likely with the use of cardioselective β-adrenoreceptor antagonists.

Key reference

Haas SJ et al. Are beta-blockers as efficacious in patients with diabetes mellitus as in patients without diabetes mellitus who have chronic heart failure? A meta-analysis of large-scale clinical trials. *Am Heart J* 2003; **146**: 848–53.

The patient with CHF and obstructive lung disease

Introduction

Obstructive lung disease is common in patients with HF, particularly those with HF of ischaemic aetiology due to the higher prevalence of smokers. It is also true that unrecognized HF exists in patients with COPD, although those with advanced lung disease often have symptoms and signs of right-ventricular failure.

The combination of HF and COPD/asthma presents particular diagnostic and therapeutic challenges:

Diagnostic
- Similar symptoms and signs.
- Poor echo windows in emphysematous patients.
- CXR—cardiothoracic ratio and evidence of pulmonary congestion unreliable in COPD.
- Assessing the severity of HF—which is the main cause of breathlessness?

Therapeutic
- Perceived contra-indication of β-adrenoreceptor antagonists.
- Difficulty assessing response to therapy.
- Significant airways disease is a relative contra-indication to cardiac transplantation.
- High diuretic dose may cause hypoventilation due to a metabolic alkalosis.
- Digoxin can cause pulmonary vasoconstriction.

Diagnosis and investigation

Patients with suspected obstructive lung disease should have spirometric pulmonary function tests performed. The stage of lung disease can then be classified by the GOLD criteria (see Table 16.1).

Other investigations indicated are those needed to confirm the presence of LVSD. These include the following:
- ECG.
- CXR.
- B-type natriuretic peptides—very useful at distinguishing between cardiac and pulmonary causes of dyspnoea.
- Echo.
- MRI/RNVG (if poor echo windows).

Table 16.1 GOLD classification of COPD

Stage	Characteristics
0: at risk	• Normal spirometry • Chronic symptoms (cough, sputum production)
I: mild COPD	• $FEV_1/FVC < 70\%$ • $FEV_1 \geq 80\%$ predicted • With or without chronic symptoms (cough, sputum production)
II: moderate COPD	• $FEV_1/FVC < 70\%$ • $30\% \leq FEV_1 < 80\%$ predicted (IIA: $50\% \leq FEV_1 < 80\%$ predicted, IIB: $30\% \leq FEV_1 < 50\%$ predicted) • With or without chronic symptoms (cough, sputum production, dyspnea)
III: severe COPD	• $FEV_1/FVC < 70\%$ • $FEV_1 < 30\%$ predicted or $FEV_1 < 50\%$ predicted plus respiratory failure or clinical signs of right heart failure

FEV_1: forced expiratory volume in 1 second; FVC: forced vital capacity; respiratory failure: arterial partial pressure of oxygen (PaO_2) <8.0kPa (60mmHg) with or without arterial partial pressure of CO_2 ($PaCO_2$) >6.7kPa (50mmHg) while breathing air at sea level. Global Initiative for Chronic Obstructive Lung Disease. National Institutes of Health. *National Heart, Lung, and Blood Institute*. Publication Number 2701. March 2001 with permission from National Heart, Lung, and Blood Institute

Treatment of CHF in COPD/asthma

ACE-inhibitor/ARBs—these may be potentially beneficial as they antagonize angiotensin-II which is a potent bronchial constrictor. They may also decrease pulmonary inflammation and vasoconstriction and thus improve alveolar membrane gas exchange.

β-adrenoreceptor antagonists—a Cochrane Review has recently shown that cardioselective β-adrenoreceptor antagonists do **not** produce adverse respiratory effects in the short term when given in mild–moderate reversible airway disease (i.e. asthma) or COPD.

▶ Given the recognized benefit of β-adrenoreceptor antagonists in heart failure, they should be administered with caution to HF patients in the presence of mild–moderate reversible airway disease or COPD.

Aldosterone antagonists—these reduce alveolar-capillary membrane damage and so may have positive effects on gas diffusion.

Digoxin—it appears that digoxin can cause pulmonary vasoconstriction, potentially adversely affecting long-term lung function, although this has not been subject to investigation.

Diuretics—standard doses of diuretics have no noticeable effect on pulmonary function, but high doses may cause hypoventilation due to a metabolic alkalosis.

Treatment of COPD/asthma in CHF

β$_2$-adrenoreceptor agonists—these are not highly selective and therefore myocardial β$_1$-receptors are often activated, causing tachycardia and increased myocardial oxygen consumption. Increased receptor stimulation may also encourage the down-regulation of these receptors and increase endogenous catecholamine production as a result.

Some studies have suggested that oral and inhaled short-acting β$_2$-adrenoreceptor agonists increase the risk of mortality and number of heart failure exacerbations in patients with left-ventricular dysfunction. The same is not thought to be true of inhaled long-acting β$_2$-adrenoreceptor agonists and therefore they are the preferred option in COPD patients with HF.

Steroids—oral steroids should be used sparingly in CHF (see p. 64).

Key references

Au DH et al. Risk of mortality and heart failure exacerbations associated with inhaled beta-adrenoceptor agonists among patients with known left ventricular systolic dysfunction. *Chest* 2003; **123**: 1964–9.

Rutten FH et al. Heart failure and chronic obstructive pulmonary disease: an ignored combination? *Eur J Heart Fail* 2006; **8**: 706–11.

Salpeter S et al. The Cochrane Library 2006, Issue 3.

Chapter 17

The patient with CHF and renal dysfunction

Introduction

Chronic heart failure is now seen not only as a cardiac disorder but rather a cardio-renal and neurohumoral syndrome.

Renal impairment is therefore common in patients with chronic heart failure. The proportion of those who have renal dysfunction increases with deteriorating NYHA functional class. A reduced glomerular filtration rate (GFR) is also associated with increased symptoms, more frequent hospitalizations and an increased mortality rate.

Definition

Serum creatinine concentration, which is often quoted as a barometer of renal impairment, is a poor indicator of renal function. Serum creatinine concentration is determined by a number of factors, other than GFR, such as gender, age, muscle mass, and ethnicity. Therefore, estimation of the GFR is preferred for the accurate assessment of renal function.

A 'normal' estimated GFR is regarded as being 120 ± 25mL/minute/ 1.73m^2 (95th centiles). Males invariably have a slightly higher GFR than females. With age, GFR tends to fall (to approximately 100mL/minute/ 1.73m^2 at age 70), although serum creatinine does not rise substantially in healthy individuals. Therefore values >90mL/minute/1.73m^2 can be regarded as normal for most patients. A GFR below 60mL/minute/1.73m^2 is associated with complications of renal disease.

Prevalence

The prevalence of renal dysfunction in CHF depends greatly on the population studied and the definition used. In the CHARM trials, the overall prevalence of a eGFR <60mL/minute/1.73m^2 was 36% (see Fig. 17.1).

Aetiology

The causes of renal impairment in CHF are multifactorial, but it is likely that the mechanisms include the following:
- Renal hypoperfusion.
- Renal artery stenosis.
- Diuretic treatment.
- Disease-modifying therapy (e.g. ACE-I, ARBs, aldosterone antagonists).
- Other concomitant medication (e.g. NSAIDs).
- Comorbidites such as diabetes and amyloid.

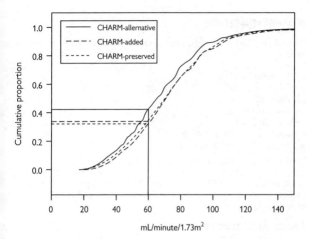

Fig. 17.1 Cumulative distribution of eGFR in patients with mild–moderate heart failure in the CHARM-preserved, CHARM-added, and CHARM-alternative trials. Reproduced from Hillege HL *et al.* Renal function as a predictor of outcome in a broad spectrum of patients with heart failure *Circulation* 2006; **113**: 671–8 with permission from Lippincott, Williams and Wilkins.

Investigations

Investigations indicated in the heart failure patient with renal dysfunction include
- U&Es.
- Diabetic screen.
- eGFR.
- Urinalysis.
- Urinary microscopy.
- Renal ultrasound.
- Auto-antibodies (e.g. ANF, ANCA).
- Very rarely, a renal biopsy.

Until recently, it was not clear how best to estimate renal function in patients with heart failure. Traditionally, eGFR was calculated by means of inulin clearance or EDTA. However, the Modification of Diet in Renal Disease (MDRD) equations have recently been validated in patients with severe CHF.

Equations to estimate GFR (expressed in mL/min/1.73m^2)

(1) MDRD-1 equation:

$$GFR = 170 \times [\text{plasma creatinine}]^{-0.999} \times [\text{age}]^{-0.176} \times [0.762 \text{ if patient is female}] \times [1.180 \text{ if patient is black}] \times [\text{SUN}]^{-0.170} \times [\text{albumin}]^{+0.318}$$

(2) MDRD-2 (abbreviated) equation:

$$GFR = 186 \times [\text{Pcr}]^{-1.154} \times [\text{age}]^{-0.203} \times [0.742 \text{ if patient is female}] \times [1.212 \text{ if patient is black}]$$

(3) Cockcroft–Gault formula normalized to a body surface area of 1.73m^2, (creatinine clearance, expressed in mL/minute/1.73m^2):

$$GFR \text{ (males)} = \frac{1.23 \times \text{weight (kg)} \times [140 - \text{age}]}{\text{plasma creatinine (μmol/L)} \times 1.73/BSA}$$

$$GFR \text{ (females)} = \frac{1.03 \times \text{weight (kg)} \times [140 - \text{age}]}{\text{plasma creatinine (μmol/L)} \times 1.73/BSA},$$

where BSA(m^2) = $\sqrt{[\text{weight (kg)} \times \text{height (cm)}/3600]}$

Prognosis

Patients with CHF and renal dysfunction have been shown to be at greater risk of mortality and morbidity, including hospitalization, independent of LVEF and NYHA class. However, a low eGFR may be a more discerning marker of an adverse prognosis in patients with non-ischaemic heart failure, compared to those with heart failure of an ischaemic aetiology (Figs. 17.2 and 17.3).

Management

- Firstly, treat any reversible causes!
- Remove/modify potentially nephrotoxic drugs, for example,
  - NSAIDs.
  - COX-2 inhibitors.
  - ACE-I.
- Multidisciplinary approach with early nephrology input.
- Dialysis where appropriate.
- Renal transplantation may be considered for patients with end-stage renal failure who develop heart failure.

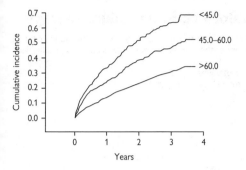

Fig. 17.2 Kaplan–Meier plot of cumulative incidence of cardiovascular death or unplanned admission to hospital for the management of worsening CHF stratified by a eGFR <45, 45–60, and >60mL/minute/1.73m^2, in patients with a LVEF <40% enrolled in the CHARM trials. Reproduced from Hillege HL *et al.* Renal function as a predictor of outcome in a broad spectrum of patients with heart failure *Circulation* 2006; **113**: 671–8 with permission from Lippincott, Williams and Wilkins.

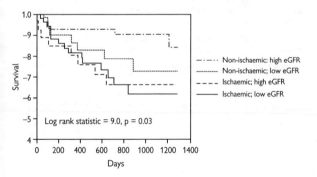

Fig. 17.3 Kaplan–Meier survival curve for eGFR in patients with ischaemic and non-ischaemic advanced heart failure. Reproduced from *Eur J Heart J* with permission from Oxford University Press.

What to do with heart failure therapy

ACE-inhibitors have been shown to provide renal protection in patients with mild–moderate and, more recently, advanced renal insufficiency. These benefits include
- Reduction in proteinuria.
- Reduction in the rate of decline of renal function.
- Delay in end-stage renal disease.
- Reduction in mortality.

In view of benefits of ACE inhibitors in both renal and heart failure, most clinicians will accept an increase in creatinine of up to 50% above baseline, or 266μmol/L (3mg/dL), whichever is the smaller, before a decision is made to reduce the dose or stop the drug, therefore careful monitoring of serum biochemistry is required.

β-adrenoreceptor antagonists The doses of bisoprolol, atenolol, and sotalol should be reduced in patients with renal dysfunction as these drugs are renally cleared (Note that the latter two drugs do not have an evidence base in CHF).

Aldosterone antagonists These should not be started in patients with a creatinine above 220μmol/L (above which patients were excluded from the trials), and the drug reduced or discontinued if creatinine rises significantly on treatment.

Digoxin The dose of digoxin will need to be reduced in renal impairment, particularly if there is electrolyte imbalance.

Furosemide Higher doses of diuretics may be needed in patients with renal impairment.

Key references

Al-Ahmad A et al. Reduced kidney function and anemia as risk factors for mortality in patients with left ventricular dysfunction. J Am Coll Cardiol 2001; **38**: 955–62.

Dries DL et al. The prognostic implications of renal insufficiency in asymptomatic and symptomatic patients with left ventricular systolic dysfunction. J Am Coll Cardiol 2000; **35**: 681–9.

Hillege HL et al. Renal function, neurohormonal activation, and survival in patients with chronic heart failure. Circulation 2000; **102**: 203–10.

Hou FF et al. Efficacy and safety of benazepril for advanced chronic renal insufficiency. N Engl J Med 2006; **354**: 131–40.

Key references

The patient with CHF and valvular heart disease

Introduction

The relation between CHF and valve disease is complex. As a consequence of left-ventricular dilatation, CHF can result in regurgitation of the mitral, aortic, or tricuspid valves.

Valve surgery may be required to improve symptoms of CHF or symptoms from the valve disease. The timing of intervention can be difficult to judge. If surgery is planned for a valvular lesion, then combining the surgery with attention to the following must be considered:

- Additional valve lesions.
- Coronary revascularization.
- Passive cardiac restraint.
- Surgery for atrial fibrillation.

The risk of operative intervention in the heart failure population should not be underestimated. The future for these patients may lie in percutaneous interventions including cardiac resynchronization or percutaneous valve replacements. There are percutaneous valves in trial for aortic stenosis, pulmonary regurgitation, and mitral regurgitation. There are also developments in percutaneous mitral annuloplasty and mitral plication.

The ACC/AHA guideline for valve disease is a very comprehensive document offering guidance in the management of patients, including those with CHF.

Key reference

Bonow RO *et al.* ACC/AHA 2006 guidelines for the management of patients with valvular heart disease. *J Am Coll Cardiol* 2006; **48**: e1–148.

Aortic valve stenosis

Aetiology

Congenital aortic stenosis (AS) is usually due to a bicuspid valve. Rheumatic AS causes fusion of the commisures and reduction in valve orifice. Degenerative AS is more common and tends to present later in life. In degenerative AS, there is annular calcification which progresses up the valve leaflets, causing an increasing limitation to flow. The underlying pathology of degenerative AS involves an inflammatory process that deposits lipids in the valve leaflets and then progresses to calcification.

Assessment

AS causes progressive obstruction of LV outflow. Therefore, the key symptoms that identify critical AS are the following:
- Exertional chest pain.
- Exertional breathlessness.
- Exertional dizziness or syncope.

The clinical signs of AS include a slow-rising carotid pulse, a harsh ejection systolic murmur that radiates to the carotids, and a quiet, single S_2.

An ECG in AS may show left-ventricular hypertrophy. Echocardiography can confirm the diagnosis, allow examination of the valve morphology, calculate valve orifice area, and quantify the gradient through the valve. Table 18.1 summarizes the echo grading of AS.

Severe AS that has caused CHF may present with a low-pressure gradient. Differentiating this scenario from CHF and incidental mild to moderate AS is difficult. In true, severe AS, the stenotic valve causes an elevated afterload, decreased ejection fraction, and low stroke volume. In CHF, contractile dysfunction results in reduced ejection fraction and low stroke volume.

▶ Further assessment is required to identify the patients who have true severe AS who may benefit from AVR. Dobutamine stress echo can be performed. Dobutamine stress echo in severe AS that will respond to surgery shows the following signs:
- Valve area will not change.
- Increase in stroke volume.
- Valve gradient increase.

Non-surgical intervention

Pharmacological methods

The inflammatory nature of degenerative AS, with its similarity to atherosclerosis, has led current investigation to focus on the role of statin therapy in slowing-down the progression of AS. Similarly, the use of ACE inhibitors, theoretically, is believed to be beneficial but small trials have given conflicting results.

Aggressive management of atrial fibrillation may be needed as the loss of atrial kick and uncontrolled ventricular rate may be disastrous to the patient's clinical condition.

Table 18.1 Echo grading of AS

	Aortic jet velocity (ms⁻¹)	Mean gradient (mmHg)	Valve area (cm²)
Normal	<1.5	<5	3.0–4.0
Mild	<3.0	<25	>1.5
Moderate	3.0–4.0	25–40	1.0–1.5
Severe	>4.0	>40	<1.0

Percutaneous intervention

In patients who are deemed unfit for AVR because of co-morbidities, consideration may be made for balloon valvotomy. Balloon valvotomy has had disappointing results because of restenosis and periprocedural complications (death 3% and MI/severe AR/myocardial perforation 6%).

Percutaneous AVR is currently a developmental technique.

Indications for surgery

The decision to proceed to AVR in a patient with severe AS and CHF relies on measurement of Doppler velocity, gradient, and valve area, and the extent of valve calcification. Severe calcification suggests that AVR may be beneficial.

The ACC/AHA guidelines for the management of patients with valvular heart disease have devised an algorithm for the management of severe AS. A modified version of this is shown in (Fig. 18.1).

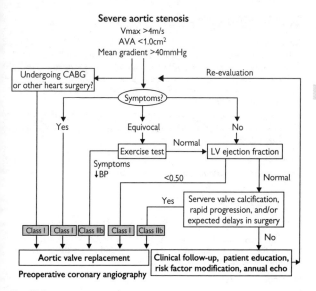

Fig. 18.1 The management of severe AS.

Key reference

Bonow RO et al. ACC/AHA 2006 guidelines for the management of patients with valvular heart disease. J Am Coll Cardiol 2006; **48**: e1–148.

Aortic regurgitation

Aetiology

Aortic regurgitation (AR) can be congenital, rheumatic, or degenerative. These usually produce chronic AR with slow, insidious LV dilation. The LV dysfunction may be reversible if AVR is performed soon after development. Chronic volume overload from AR may cause irreversible LV dysfunction even after AVR.

Acute severe AR may be caused by infective endocarditis, aortic dissection, or trauma and can result in catastrophic elevation of LV filling pressures and heart failure.

Assessment

The key symptoms that suggest severe AR include
- Angina.
- Breathlessness.
- Symptoms of CHF.

Clinical signs include collapsing pulses and an early diastolic murmur.

The ECG may show left-ventricular hypertrophy. Echocardiography can confirm the diagnosis, determine the severity, and assess the LV systolic function (Table 18.2).

Non-surgical intervention

Pharmacological methods

There is trial evidence that supports the use of vasodilators, specifically nifedipine, to slow-down progression of AR. However, the presence of CHF would discourage the use of nifedipine.

Indications for surgery

Approximately 15% of valves can be repaired rather than replaced. Again a modified version of the ACC/AHA algorithm is illustrated in Fig 18.2.

Table 18.2 Echo grading of AR

	Mild AR	Severe AR
Jet width (% of LVOT)	<25%	>60%
Vena contracta width	<0.3cm	>0.6cm
Pressure half-time	>500ms	<200ms
LV size	Normal	Dilated

Chronic severe aortic regurgitation

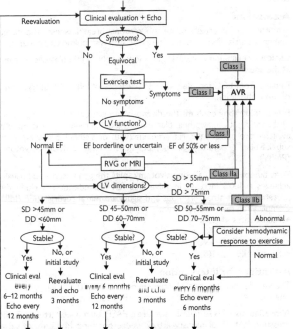

Fig. 18.2 The management of chronic severe AR.

Key references

Bonow RO et al. ACC/AHA 2006 guidelines for the management of patients with valvular heart disease. *J Am Coll Cardiol* 2006; **48**: e1–148.

Bekeredjian R & Grayburn PA. Valvular heart disease: aortic regurgitation. *Circulation* 2005; **112**: 125–34.

Mitral stenosis

Aetiology

The vast majority mitral of stenosis (MS) is due to rheumatic heart disease. There are a small number of cases attributable to congenital valve disease. Other rare causes include carcinoid disease (almost always in conjunction with an atrial right-to-left shunt, e.g. patent foramen ovale) and connective tissue diseases such as rheumatoid arthritis and systemic lupus erythematosis.

MS is associated with right-heart failure and pulmonary hypertension. LV systolic function is usually preserved. Chronic afterload elevation and preload reduction causes reduced LV systolic function in about 25% of cases.

Assessment

Symptoms of MS usually relate to exertional breathlessness. The development of atrial fibrillation may be associated with pulmonary oedema.

Clinical examination demonstrates a low, rumbling mid-diastolic murmur at the apex.

Findings from ECG include p mitrale (evidence of left atrial enlargement) or atrial fibrillation.

Echocardiography confirms the diagnosis and can determine the severity of the lesion. It can also help plan the possible interventions. The options available are mitral valve replacement (with or without preservation of sub-valvular apparatus) or percutaneous mitral balloon valvotomy (PMBV).

Percutaneous mitral balloon valvotomy splits the commisures and usually achieves a 100% increase in valve area. Contra-indications include the presence of left-atrial thrombus and significant mitral regurgitation (MR). Complication rates are significant:
- Failure rates 1–15%
- Death 0–3%
- Embolism 0.5–5%
- Severe MR 2–10%.

Indications for intervention

The key decider in terms of intervention is the patient's functional class. The ACC/AHA guidelines are shown in (Figs 18.3 and 18.4).

Abbreviations—MVA: mitral valve area; PASP: pulmonary artery systolic pressure; PAWP: pulmonary artery wedge pressure; MVG: mean valve gradient; PMBV: percutaneous mitral valve valvotomy; MVR: mitral valve replacement.

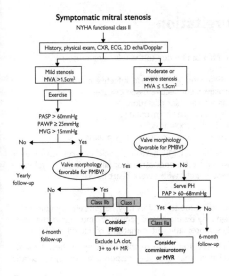

Fig. 18.3 MS and NYHA functional class II.

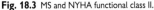

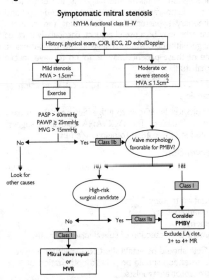

Fig. 18.4 MS and NYHA functional class III–IV.

Mitral regurgitation

Aetiology

Mitral regurgitation (MR) can be due to the following causes:
- Primary valve disease.
  - For example, rheumatic heart disease, infective endocarditis, mitral valve prolapse, connective tissue disease.
- Functional secondary to annular dilatation.
  - For example, ischaemic cardiomyopathy.
- Failure of the mitral valve apparatus.
  - For example, rupture chordae or papillary muscle.

The majority of patients with MR have a chronic progression of their symptoms. Those with infective endocarditis or failure of the mitral valve apparatus may present acutely, with severe heart failure.

Assessment

Patients with mild or even moderate MR may be entirely asymptomatic. The only physical sign may be the classic pansystolic murmur at the apex. Severe MR is usually symptomatic with symptoms of left-sided CHF.

An ECG is helpful in establishing the rhythm, as many of these patients develop atrial fibrillation that may be responsible for symptomatic deterioration.

Trans-thoracic echocardiography confirms the diagnosis and documents the severity of the lesion. Echo can also help define the aetiology and consider whether pulmonary hypertension is developing (an ominous sign). Trans-oesophageal echo may be a useful adjunct, particularly in cases with symptomatic change without obvious change in the trans-thoracic echo assessment. Some of these patients may be found to have severe MR on trans-oesophageal studies.

Further assessment of MR can be made with cardiac catheterization or magnetic resonance scanning.

The severity of MR is notoriously difficult to judge. Severe MR is usually associated with left-atrial dilatation. The ACC/AHA guidelines suggest the features demonstrated in (Table 18.3) to help grade MR.

Indications for intervention

At present there are five different possible interventions for patients with MR and CHF:
1. Pharmacology.
2. Cardiac resynchronization therapy.
3. Mitral valve repair ± annuloplasty.
4. Mitral valve replacement.
5. Mitral valve replacement and resection of subvalvular apparatus.

Patients with MR and CHF should be established on maximum tolerated CHF therapy. Particular attention should be paid to optimization of ACE inhibitor and β-adrenoreceptor antagonists.

Table 18.3 ACC/AHA classification of MR severity

	Mitral Regurgitation		
	Mild	**Moderate**	**Severe**
Qualitative			
Angiographic grade	1+	2+	3–4+
Color Doppler jet area	Small, central jet (<4cm^2 or <20% LA area)	Signs of MR greater than mild present but no criteria for severe MR	Vena contracta width greater than 0.7cm with large central MR jet (area >40% of LA area) or with a wall-impinging jet of any size, swirling in LA
Doppler vena contracta width (cm)	<0.3	0.3–0.69	≥0.70
Quantitative (cath or echo)			
Regurgitant volume (mL per beat)	<30	30–59	≥60
Regurgitant fraction (%)	<30	30–49	≥50
Regurgitant orifice area (cm^2)	<0.20	0.2–0.39	≥0.40
Additional essential criteria			
Left atrial size			Enlarged
Left ventricular size			Enlarged

There is a small body of evidence considering the role of cardiac resynchronization therapy. LV dyssynchrony including the posterior mitral leaflet is important in the aetiology of mitral regurgitation. Cardiac resynchronization therapy may improve mitral regurgitation by restoring synchronous LV contraction acutely, and further improvements may be achieved by ventricular remodelling.

Whether performed in isolation or in addition to coronary revascularization or more novel techniques such as passive cardiac restraint (e.g. CorCap), MV surgery can achieve significant improvements in symptoms of CHF. However, the significant morbidity and mortality of cardiac surgery in this patient group with severe MR and CHF should not be underestimated.

There is an increasing body of evidence supporting MV repair as the operation of choice when technically feasible. This evidence is from patients with ischaemic and non-ischaemic cardiomyopathies. Mitral valve repair achieves beneficial effects of restoring the MV architecture and competence, without challenging the ventricle with a fully competent prosthetic valve replacement. This can be combined with annuloplasty to further improve the MV architecture.

The ACC/AHA guidelines from 2006 have described clinical settings in which MV repair is appropriate but MV replacement is not (Fig. 18.5).

The subvalvular apparatus is well established in its importance in LV function after MV replacement. The MV apparatus achieves continuity between mitral annulus and left-ventricular free wall through the chordae and papillary muscles. The subvalvular apparatus is therefore preserved unless it is so diseased that it must be resected. There are now prosthetic options that may facilitate repair of the apparatus.

Mitral valve surgery may be combined with surgery for atrial fibrillation. There are a variety of techniques including the Maze procedure and radiofrequency ablation devices.

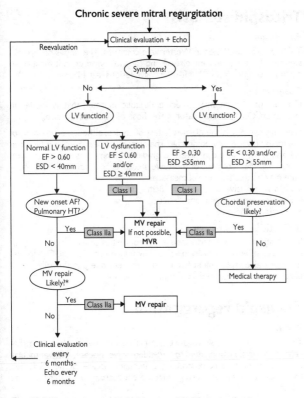

Fig. 18.5 The management of chronic severe MR. EF: ejection fraction; ESD: end-systolic diameter; HT: hypertension.

Key reference

Bax JJ & Poldermans D. Mitral regurgitation and left ventricular dyssynchrony: implications for treatment. *Heart* 2006; **92**: 1363–64.

Tricuspid stenosis

Aetiology

This is a rare valve lesion in Westernized countries. The causes of tricuspid stenosis (TS) are rheumatic disease and carcinoid syndrome. It most often occurs in conjunction with left-sided valve lesions, e.g. MS.

Assessment

Careful auscultation may detect a diastolic murmur that is louder in inspiration. Other clinical features are those of right-heart failure.

Echocardiography is the diagnostic test of choice, although assessment of the tricuspid valve may be difficult. The normal TV peak E wave is between 0.3 and 0.7m/s. A mean pressure gradient >5mmHg is consistent with severe TS. Measurement of the valve area is difficult and pressure –half-time may be the most useful measure.

- Normal TV valve area $7–8cm^2$
- Develop pressure gradient $<2cm^2$
- Develop symptoms $<1.5cm^2$

Indications for surgery

Intervention is usually performed in the context of other valve surgery. In rare cases of pure TS, balloon valvotomy may be considered. Otherwise, tricuspid valve replacement is the most frequent operation usually with a bioprosthetic valve to reduce the thrombotic risk.

Tricuspid regurgitation

Aetiology

The majority of tricuspid regurgitation (TR) is functional, related to right-ventricular dysfunction, due to left-sided valve disease, left-ventricular dysfunction, or chronic obstructive pulmonary disease. Some TR is due to primary valve disease such as infective endocarditis or rheumatic heart disease.

Assessment

Symptoms are usually those of right-heart failure. Signs include a pansystolic murmur accentuated by inspiration, a raised JVP and tender, pulsatile hepatomegaly.

Echocardiography confirms the diagnosis and the severity. Severe TR is associated with:
- Regurgitant volume >45ml.
- Effective regurgitant orifice area $>40mm^2$.

Indications for intervention

Intervention is usually considered at the time of intervention for left-sided valve lesions. TV repair can occasionally be performed. Increasingly TV annuloplasty is the intervention of choice for functional TR. In primary valve disease, TVR may be required. This carries a high operative morality of between 7 and 40%.

Key reference

Tang GH *et al.* Tricuspid valve repair with an annuloplasty ring results in improved long-term outcomes. *Circulation* 2006; **114**(Suppl 1): I577–81.

Pulmonary stenosis

Aetiology

The majority of pulmonary stenosis (PS) occurs as congenital heart disease in isolation or as a component of tetralogy of Fallot or Noonan's syndrome. In adults, few patients have symptomatic PS as it is usually mild or moderate, and related to thickening and doming of a morphologically normal valve in the absence of calcification.

Assessment

Symptoms are usually mild and include breathlessness, progressing to right-heart failure. Signs include an ejection systolic murmur in the pulmonary region, augmented by inspiration.

Echocardiography confirms the diagnosis and severity:
- Mild PS   <3m/s
- Moderate PS   3–4m/s
- Severe PS   >4m/s.

Cardiac catheterization is indicated if the transvalvular gradient is >3m/s.

Indications for surgery

Percutaneous balloon valvotomy is recommended in symptomatic patients with a gradient >30mmHg, or in asymptomatic patients with a gradient >40mmHg. Pulmonary valve replacement is reserved for patients with a severely dysplastic valve.

Pulmonary regurgitation

Aetiology

Significant pulmonary regurgitation (PR) essentially only occurs in patients with congenital heart disease, e.g. following repair of tetralogy of Fallot. Occasional acquired cases of PR may be the result of infective endocarditis or carcinoid syndrome.

Assessment

Significant PR may present with symptoms of right-heart failure, CHF, or arrhythmias. The murmur is an early diastolic murmur in the pulmonary region accentuated by inspiration.

Echocardiography confirms the diagnosis and the severity of the lesion. Severe PR is defined as the colour flow map of PR filling the RV outflow tract and a dense continuous wave Doppler signal with a short pressure half-time (<90ms).

Indications for surgery

In tetralogy of Fallot, a QRS duration >180ms has been shown to correlate with RV size and predicts malignant ventricular arrhythmias and sudden death. Pulmonary valve replacement (PVR) has been shown to reduce RV end-diastolic volume.

PVR is considered in NYHA II or III with severe PR. In asymptomatic patients, the timing of PVR remains unclear.

Key reference

Davlouros PA *et al.* Timing and type of surgery for severe pulmonary regurgitation after repair of tetralogy of Fallot. *Int J Cardiol* 2004; 97: 91–101.

Chapter 19

The patient with CHF and specific heart muscle disease

Introduction

Cardiomyopathies are diseases of heart muscle (Fig. 19.1). In 1995, the WHO/International Society and Federation of Cardiology Task Force on the Definition and Classification of the Cardiomyopathies defined cardiomyopathies as 'diseases of the myocardium associated with cardiac dysfunction' and classified them into the following types:

- Dilated cardiomyopathy.
- Hypertrophic cardiomyopathy.
- Restrictive cardiomyopathy.
- Arrhythmogenic right ventricular cardiomyopathy.
- Unclassified cardiomyopathies (e.g. LV non-compaction).

Dilated cardiomyopathy

There are many known causes of dilated cardiomyopathy, and they can be further classified according to their aetiology into:

- Ischaemic (📖 Chapter 10).
- Valvular (📖 Chapter 18).
- Familial.
- Hypertensive.
- Metabolic and nutritional.
- Inflammatory—as a consequence of myocarditis.
- Muscular dystrophies.
- Neuromuscular disorders.
- Systemic disease.
- Peripartum.
- Toxic—for example chemotherapy agents (📖 discussed further in Chapter 22) and alcohol.

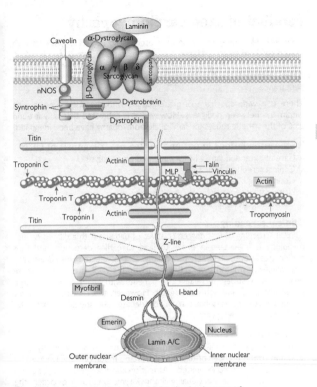

Fig. 19.1 Proteins and pathways involved in the development of cardiomyopathies. MLP, muscle LIM protein; nNOS, neuronal nitric oxide synthase. Reproduced from Towbin JA & Bowles NE. *The failing heart*. Nature 2002; **415**: 227–33 with permission from Nature Publishing Group.

Familial dilated cardiomyopathy

A familial link is now known to be present in up to 50% of patients with dilated cardiomyopathy. Numerous gene mutations have been identified, the majority of which are in the genes coding for cytoskeletal proteins. Approximately 90% of mutations are autosomal dominant with variable penetrance.

There is a wide spectrum of presentations with the phenotype varying within and between pedigrees. However, it is estimated that only around 25% of the genetic causes for familial cardiomyopathy have been identified.

Recommendations in patients with a new diagnosis of DCM

- Careful extended family history and pedigree analysis.
- Clinical screening of first degree relatives.
- Counselling of at-risk family members.
- Liaise with a geneticist.
- Consider genetic testing.

Clinical screening

Clinical screening of first degree relatives of patients with a dilated cardiomyopathy is important in order to lead to earlier detection, and thus earlier treatment, of LVSD, particularly as the affected individuals may not manifest symptoms of CHF or arrhythmias until late in the disease process. All first-degree relatives of patients with DCM should undergo a periodic ECG and echocardiogram. However, the required frequency of such screening is subject to much debate, but should probably be performed every 3–5 years.

Genetic testing and counselling

Genetic testing for familial cardiomyopathy is not currently widely available due to the number of different genes and mutations involved (Table 19.1). It can provide only limited information about an inherited condition and not whether an individual will show symptoms of a disorder, the severity of the symptoms, or its natural history.

Genetic testing must begin with an affected family member in order for the testing to be useful, and only if a causative mutation is identified is it possible to offer informative testing to at-risk relatives. However, excluding the mutation in an at-risk family member can be extremely reassuring and avoid the need for periodic clinical screening.

Table 19.1 Mutations identified and their frequency in familial dilated and hypertrophic cardiomyopathy

Protein	Gene	Transmission	Mutation frequency (%)	Association with HCM?
β-myosin heavy chain	MYH7	AD	5–10	Yes
Lamin A/C	LMNA	AD	5–10	
Cardiac troponin T	TNNT2	AD	2–4	Yes
Cypher/LIM	ZASP/LBD3	AD	2–4	
Cardiac sodium channel	SCN5A	AD	2–4	
Metavinculin	VCL	AD	1	
α-Tropomyosin	TPM1	AD	<1	Yes
Thymopoietin	TMPO	AD	<1	
SUR2A	ABCC	AD	<1	
Muscle LIM protein	CSRP3	AD	<1	
α-actinin 2	ACTN2	AD	<1	
Telethonin	TCAP	AD	<1	
Actin	ACTC	AD	<<1	Yes
Delta sarcoglycan	SGCD	AD	<<1	
Cardiac troponin C	TNNC1	AD	<<1	Yes
Desmin	DES	AD	<<1	
α-myosin heavy chain	MHY6	AD	Unknown	Yes
Phospholamban	PLN	AD	Unknown	
Myosin binding protein C	MYBPC	AD	Unknown	Yes
Eyes absent 4	EYA4	AD	Unknown	
Titin	TTN	AD	Unknown	Yes
Dystrophin	DMD	X-linked	Unknown	
Tafazzin	TAZ/G4.5	X-linked	Unknown	
Cardiac troponin I	TNNI3	AR	<1	Yes

Key reference
Burkett EL & Hershberger RE. Clinical and genetic issues in familial dilated cardiomyopathy. *J Am Coll Cardiol* 2005; **45**: 969–81.

Hypertensive cardiomyopathy

Hypertensive cardiomyopathy is the most common cause of chronic heart failure outside the Western world. Hypertension causes left ventricular hypertrophy as a compensatory mechanism to an increased after-load, by normalizing systolic wall stress and preserving contractile function. However, the failure of further hypertrophy to normalize loading conditions results in progressive cardiac dysfunction and dilatation, as well as interstitial and perivascular fibrosis.

Cardiomyocyte apoptosis has also been shown to be abnormally stimulated in the hypertrophied heart of patients with hypertension. This process is increased further in those who develop chronic heart failure, and therefore apoptosis may be one of the many mechanisms involved in the loss of contractile mass and function in hypertensive cardiomyopathy (see Fig. 19.2).

Metabolic cardiomyopathy

Metabolic cardiomyopathies are generally caused by an underlying deficiency of energy production due to a wide variety of defects, including glycolipid, fatty acid, and glucose metabolism. Of these, Fabry and Pompe disease are discussed in more detail on 📖 pp. 266 and 264. Other metabolic cardiomyopathies include
- Carnitine deficiency.
- Mitochondrial myopathies.

General system disease

Cardiac involvement is recognized in general system disease, particularly autoimmune diseases. Systemic lupus erythematosis, for example, causes a pancarditis in approximately 10% of patients involving the pericardium, myocardium, endocardium, and coronary arteries, although patients may be asymptomatic.

Neuromuscular disorders

Cardiac involvement commonly occurs in Friedreich's ataxia, although this is usually asymptomatic. It is much more likely to be associated with HCM, rather than DCM.

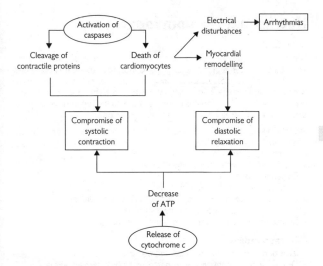

Fig. 19.2 Mechanisms activated by the apoptotic process in the cardiomyocyte that may contribute to a deterioration of cardiac function and alter the electrical activity of the myocardium in hypertensive cardiomyopathy. Cytochrome c plays a major role in ATP production through mitochondrial oxidative phosphorylation. Caspases are proteases involved in the execution of the apoptotic process. Reproduced from Gonzalez A et al. Cardiomyocyte apoptosis in hypertensive cardiomyopathy. *Cardiovasc Res* 2003; **59**: 549–62 with permission from Elsevier.

Nutritional cardiomyopathy

Beri-beri

Beri-beri is caused by a deficiency in thiamine (vitamin B_1), which is an important co-enzyme in the hexose monophosphate shunt. It is prevalent in Asia where the diet consists of large quantities of polished rice, which is deficient in thiamine, and initially presents as a high-output cardiac failure. Beri-beri can less commonly develop in patients on chronic diuretic therapy, due to increased urinary thiamine excretion.

Seven diagnostic criteria for classic beri-beri heart disease have been proposed:
- ≥3 months of thiamine-deficient diet.
- Cardiomegaly, with normal sinus rhythm.
- Dependent oedema.
- Signs of neuritis, pellagra, or both.
- Minor ECG changes (e.g. non-specific ST/T abnormalities).
- No other identifiable cause for heart disease.
- Response to thiamine therapy or autopsy evidence.

Clinical features
- Wet beri-beri—fatigue, malaise, and oedema.
- Dry beri-beri—peripheral neuropathy, and a high cardiac output.
- Anaemia (if there is coexisting iron or folate deficiency).
- Painful glossitis.
- Hyperkeratinized skin lesions.
- Reduced thiamine, increased serum pyruvate and lactate, low red cell transketolase.

Treatment
Thiamine—the initial loading doses of thiamine are 100–500mg intravenously, followed by 25–100mg/day orally for at least 2 weeks. Patients often have a prompt improvement in cardiac function.

Other nutritional cardiomyopathies
Deficiencies in certain other micro- and macro-nutrients (e.g. selenium and zinc) have been implicated in the development of DCM. However, due to the complex individual diets in those with a non-ischaemic cardiomyopathy, this is usually impossible to unravel, and even more difficult to study!

Peripartum cardiomyopathy

Peripartum cardiomyopathy (PPCM) is a rare disorder where LVSD occurs between the last month of pregnancy and 5-months post-partum. A similar condition has been recognized in earlier pregnancy, but it is uncertain whether this is part of the same entity, or whether pregnancy has unmasked pre-existing cardiac dysfunction. In either case, it is important to exclude other causes of cardiomyopathy.

Several mechanisms for PPCM have been investigated, including nutritional disorders (e.g. selenium deficiency), autoimmune disease, myocarditis, abnormal hormonal regulation, viral triggers, and fetal microchimerism (fetal cells in maternal blood) causing the initiation of an autoimmune myocarditis. However, the aetiology remains unknown.

Possible risk factors for PPCM include
- Extremes of childbearing age.
- Multiparity.
- African origin.
- Toxaemia.
- Hypertension of pregnancy.
- Use of tocolytics (medications used to suppress premature labour).
- Multiple pregnancy.

Clinical features
- Symptoms and signs of HF (may initially be masked by pregnancy).
- Hypodynamic apical impulse.
- S_3 gallop.
- ECG—non-specific ST/T abnormalities are seen in the majority of cases; LVH by electrical criteria in two-thirds.
- Echo—dilated LV with LVSD; thrombus may be present.

Treatment
Standard HF therapy is indicated in PPCM following childbirth. In particular, β-adrenoreceptor antagonists are important in order to reduce the risks of arrhythmia and sudden death.

However, ACE inhibitors are known to be teratogenic and should therefore be replaced by hydralazine and nitrates, at least until delivery.

Prognosis
Women with PPCM have a higher rate of spontaneous recovery of ventricular function than those with other forms of DCM. This usually occurs in the first 6 months, although can take significantly longer than this. However, PPCM is still associated with a mortality of approximately 15%. For some, ventricular assist devices or cardiac transplantation becomes necessary—occasionally requiring urgent listing.

Subsequent pregnancy
There is a significant risk for recurrence or death during subsequent pregnancies, particularly if cardiac function has not returned to normal first. Patients should therefore be advised against further pregnancy.

Key reference

Sliwa K, Fett J & Elkayam U. Peripartum cardiomyopathy. *Lancet* 2006; **368**: 687–93.

Alcoholic cardiomyopathy

Chronic excessive alcohol consumption is a leading secondary cause of non-ischaemic cardiomyopathy. The majority of cases appear to be related to the direct toxic effect of alcohol on myocardial function, although nutritional deficiency (e.g. beri-beri) and additives to alcohol (e.g. cobalt) have also been implicated in a minority of cases.

Up to one-third of alcoholics have evidence of LVSD. However, not all alcoholics develop cardiomyopathy as there appears to be a genetic predisposition to its development: those with a DD phenotype of the ACE gene polymorphism are significantly more likely to develop LVSD than those without. It is important to emphasize that recovery of cardiac function can occur if the disease is diagnosed early and further alcohol intake halted.

Clinical features
- History of chronic alcohol excess.
- Symptoms and signs of a dilated cardiomyopathy of any aetiology.
- Atrial fibrillation is a relatively common finding.
- Possible signs of coexisting alcoholic liver disease.

Treatment
- Complete abstinence from alcohol.
- Standard CHF therapy.
- Vitamin supplementation (e.g. thiamine, folate).

Tachycardiomyopathy

Incessant tachycardia is a recognized cause of non-ischaemic cardiomyopathy. Indeed, atrial fibrillation, atrial flutter, ectopic atrial tachycardia, atrioventricular tachycardia (AVRT), atrioventricular nodal tachycardia (AVNRT), and ventricular tachycardia have all been shown to cause such a *tachycardiomyopathy*. Although the rate of the tachycardia appears to correlate with the degree of LVSD, the mechanism for myocardial dysfunction is not clear. However, as arrhythmias are frequently the result of cardiomyopathy, they are easily overlooked as the potential cause. Importantly, though, definitive treatment of the arrhythmia can result in complete reversal of the myocardial dysfunction.

The muscular dystrophies

There are a number of inherited progressive myopathic disorders that are associated with cardiac involvement. They include
- Duchenne muscular dystrophy (DMD).
- Becker muscular dystrophy (BMD).
- Myotonic dystrophy.

The dystrophinopathies

Both Duchenne and Becker muscular dystrophies are X-linked recessive disorders of the dystrophin gene. DMD is more common than BMD, with an incidence of approximately 1 in 3500 male births compared with 1 in 30 000 male births. Proximal muscle weakness is the predominant symptom in both conditions, and the development of a cardiomyopathy with conduction abnormalities and arrhythmias is well recognized (although less common in BMD). In general, DMD presents earlier, and has a more severe course, than BMD.

Clinical findings
- Pseudohypertrophy of the calf.
- Lumbar lordosis.
- Waddling gait.
- Shortening of the Achilles tendons.
- Hyporeflexia or areflexia.

Investigations
- Elevated creatine kinase (10–20 × normal).
- Electromyography—myopathic changes.
- Electrocardiogram—tall right pre-cordial R waves with an increased R/S ratio and deep Q waves in lateral leads. Also associated with conduction disturbances.
- Muscle biopsy.
- Dystrophin analysis—marked reduction in dystrophin (DMD) or abnormal molecular weight (BMD).
- Genetic analysis.

Treatment
- Supportive.
- Standard CHF therapy in those with a cardiomyopathy.
- Consider PPM/CRT in those with conduction abnormalities.

Myotonic dystrophy

Myotonic dystrophy is an autosomal dominant disorder of the myotonin gene affecting 1:20 000 people. Myotonin is a protein kinase that transfers phosphate from ATP to other enzymes, and thus is involved in a diverse array of biochemical processes.

Symptoms typically occur in adolescence or adulthood, and include weakness and wasting affecting facial muscles, arms, and legs. Myotonia (delayed muscle relaxation after contraction), cataracts, and abnormal intellectual functioning are also the other features. Around 10% develop a cardiomyopathy, caused by myocardial fatty infiltration, fibrosis, and atrophy of the cardiac conduction system. Such patients are at risk of sudden death due to conductive system disease. However, the main cause of death is respiratory failure.

Investigations

- Electromyography (EMG).
- Mildly elevated serum CK concentration.
- Muscle biopsy.
- ECG—the presence of pathologic Q waves in the absence of coronary artery disease is an indicator of myocardial involvement.
  ▶ Beware of conduction system disease, which can progress rapidly.
- Echocardiography.
- Genetic testing—CTG trinucleotide repeat.

Treatment

- Supportive (no specific therapy).
- Standard CHF therapy in those with a cardiomyopathy.
- Consider PPM/CRT in those with conduction abnormalities—patients should undergo yearly ECGs, or more frequently if conduction system involvement suspected.

Fabry disease

Fabry disease is an X-linked recessive glycolipid storage disease. It is caused by deficient activity of the lysosomal enzyme, α-galactosidase A, which results in the progressive accumulation of globotriaosylceramide in the vascular system, renal epithelial cells, myocardial cells, dorsal root ganglia, and autonomic nervous system.

The incidence of Fabry disease is estimated to be 1:40 000. Expression of the clinical phenotype in heterozygous female carriers varies, with some females exhibiting severe signs of the disease because of random X-chromosome inactivation.

Clinical features

Clinical manifestations are invariably evident by 10 years of age, and initially include:
- Angiokeratomas in the groin, hips, and umbilical region.
- Peripheral neuropathy (with normal nerve conduction studies).
- Asymptomatic corneal dystrophy.

With advancing age, other disease becomes increasingly important:
- Cardiac involvement.
  - Cardiomyopathy.
  - Conduction disease.
  - Myocardial infarction secondary to the accumulation of lipids moieties in angiographically normal coronary arteries.
  - Valvular defects—for example aortic stenosis and mitral regurgitation.
- Cerebrovascular disease leading to aneurysms, acute blindness, and stroke.
- Renal disease—initially evident as proteinuria, often progresses to renal failure by the time the patient reaches 30–40 years of age.

Investigation

There is a reduced or absent α-galactosidase A activity in plasma or peripheral leukocytes in affected males. Carriers may have a normal enzyme activity and therefore this assay is not reliable, and potential carriers should undergo molecular studies to detect the family's mutation.

Treatment

No cure exists for Fabry disease, although enzyme replacement with recombinant human α-galactosidase A has recently been approved for use. However, important questions regarding optimal dosing and long-term benefits remain to be answered. Standard heart failure therapy should be initiated in Fabry patients with cardiomyopathy, and other treatment directed against specific manifestations of the disease.

A Fabry disease registry has been established to better understand the variability and progression of the disease—www.fabryregistry.com

Pompe disease

Pompe disease is an autosomal recessive glycogen storage disorder that results in a deficiency of acid α-glucosidase, a lysosomal enzyme that hydrolyzes lysosomal glycogen to glucose. The accumulation of glycogen in certain tissues, especially muscles, impairs their ability to function normally and therefore muscle weakness is a prominent feature in all forms of Pompe disease.

Pompe disease is an extremely heterogeneous disorder that varies with respect to age at onset, rate of disease progression, and extent of organ involvement, with infantile-onset disease progressing much more rapidly than adult-onset disease and ultimately proves fatal, usually within the first year of life. It is thought to affect around 1 in 40 000 people.

Clinical features

The following are the features of adult-onset disease:
- Progressive proximal muscle weakness and exercise intolerance.
- Gait abnormalities.
- Hypotonia.
- Respiratory insufficiency.
- Sleep apnoea.
- Restrictive and dilated cardiomyopathies (rare in adult-onset disease).

Investigation

The definitive test is the measurement of acid α-glucosidase, with muscle and skin fibroblasts providing the most reliable results. Genotyping is important in genetic counselling and may be of supportive diagnostic value.

Treatment

Pompe disease leads to progressive muscular degeneration and premature death. There is no cure for Pompe disease, and treatment has largely been limited to supportive care. However, in 2006, the FDA approved enzyme replacement therapy with alglucosidase alfa (rhGAA) as an option for treating Pompe disease, although trial experience is currently limited to two small studies of infantile-onset disease.

Cardiac sarcoid

Sarcoidosis is a multi-system, non-caseating, granulomatous disease of unknown aetiology. It is estimated to affect 1:10 000 people, with marked geographical and racial variation, being three to four times more common in blacks. It typically affects young adults, and usually presents with either evidence of bilateral hilar lymphadenopathy or pulmonary infiltrates, or skin or eye lesions.

Sarcoidosis most commonly affects the lung. Cardiac involvement is uncommon, affecting only around 2–5% of patients with sarcoidosis, although autopsy studies indicate that sub-clinical cardiac involvement is more common (Fig. 19.3).

Pathophysiology

The aetiology of sarcoidosis is not clear. Several potential antigens have been suggested as triggers, including *Mycobacterium tuberculosis*, Mycoplasma species, aluminium, and pollen. T-helper cell activation leads to the formation of granuloma lesion, and interleukin-6 is thought to be involved in the maintenance of inflammation by inducing T cell proliferation. A positive association with cardiac sarcoidosis has been reported with HLA-DQB1*0601.

Clinical features

The clinical sequelae of cardiac sarcoidosis range from asymptomatic conduction abnormalities to fatal ventricular arrhythmias, depending upon the location and extent of granulomatous inflammation.

Cardiac manifestations include
- Complete heart block.
- Other conduction abnormalities.
- Ventricular tachycardia.
- Supraventricular arrhythmias (e.g. re-entrant tachyarrhythmias, atrial flutter, fibrillation, and tachycardia).
- Congestive heart failure.
- Pericardial effusion (rarely causing tamponade).
- Constrictive pericarditis.
- Valvular dysfunction (including mitral valve prolapse).

Prognosis

Most patients with cardiac sarcoidosis ultimately die from ventricular tachyarrhythmia, conduction disturbances, or progressive heart failure.

Guidelines for the diagnosis of cardiac sarcoidosis based on the Study Report on Diffuse Pulmonary Diseases From the Japanese Ministry of Health and Welfare, 1993

1. Histologic diagnosis group: endomyocardial biopsy demonstrates epithelioid granulomata without caseating granulomata.
2. Clinical diagnosis group: in patients with histologic diagnosis of extracardiac sarcoidosis, cardiac sarcoidosis is suspected when 'a' and at least one of the criteria 'b' to 'e' is present, and other aetiologies such as hypertension and coronary artery disease have been excluded:
   a. Complete RBBB, left-axis deviation, AV block, VT, PVC, or pathological Q or ST-T change on resting or ambulatory electrocardiogram.
   b. Abnormal wall motion, regional wall thinning, or dilation of the left ventricle.
   c. Perfusion defect by ^{201}Tl-myocardial scintigraphy or abnormal accumulation by ^{67}Ga-citrate or ^{99}Tc-PYP myocardial scintigraphy.
   d. Abnormal intracardiac pressure, low cardiac output, or abnormal wall motion or depressed ejection fraction of the left ventricle.
   e. Interstitial fibrosis or cellular infiltration over moderate grade even if the findings are non-specific VT, ventricular tachycardia.

Key reference

Hiraga H et al. The Japanese Ministry of Health and Welfare, 1993; 23–4.

Investigations

The clinical findings of cardiac sarcoidosis are largely non-specific. As a result, diagnostic tests such as myocardial biopsy may be required, particularly in patients without other manifestations of sarcoidosis.

- Serum ACE.
- Kveim–Siltzbach test.
- Electrocardiography.
- 24-hour Holter monitoring.
- CXR.
- Echocardiography—the ventricular septum often appears hyperechogenic; evidence of LVSD or LV aneurysm.
- Endomyocardial biopsy (Fig. 19.3) —however, myocardial involvement can be patchy and more commonly occur basally, whereas endomyocardial biopsy specimens are usually obtained from the apical septum.
- Nuclear imaging—particularly Thallium-201 scintigraphy.
- Magnetic resonance imaging.
- Coronary angiography.

Treatment

Corticosteroids are thought capable of halting or slowing the progression of inflammation and fibrosis in sarcoidosis. The initial starting dose is 60–80mg of prednisone daily, with a gradual tapering of the dose to a maintenance level of 10–15mg per day over a period of 6 months. Cushingoid side-effects are most common in doses over 7.5mg. However, a possible association between corticosteroid treatment and formation of ventricular aneurysms has been described. Alternative agents such as chloroquine, hydroxychloroquine, and methotrexate may be given to patients who do not respond to corticosteroids or who cannot tolerate their side-effects.

A permanent pacemaker is indicated in patients with complete heart block or other high-grade conduction system disease. An ICD is recommended in survivors of sudden death or patients with refractory ventricular tachyarrhythmias. Some also recommend an ICD for primary prevention due to the high rate of sudden death due to ventricular tachyarrhythmias in cardiac sarcoidosis.

Cardiac transplantation for cardiac sarcoidosis is rare. It remains, however, a possibility for younger patients with severe end-stage irreversible cardiac failure or resistant VT, although recurrent disease in the transplanted heart can occur. Other types of surgery may be occasionally required, such as correction of mitral valve disease or resection of ventricular aneurysms.

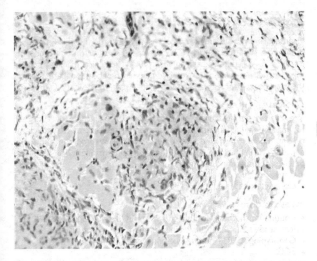

Fig. 19.3 (See colour plate 2) Sarcoidosis. A central non-caseating granuloma is disrupting the myocardium with myocyte destruction and early replacement fibrosis. A second granuloma is present at the bottom left. Haematoxylin and eosin ×400. Courtesy of Dr Allan McPhaden, Glasgow Royal Infirmary.

Key reference

Baughman RP. Clinical characteristics of patients in a case control study of sarcoidosis. *Am J Resp Crit Care Med* 2001; **164**: 1885–9.

Haemochromatosis

Haemochromatosis is an autosomal recessive disorder in which mutations in the HFE gene (particularly C282Y—on the short arm of chromosome 6) cause increased intestinal iron absorption. The clinical manifestations of this disorder are related to excessive tissue iron deposition, particularly in the liver, heart, pancreas, and pituitary, but also in the heart (Fig. 19.4).

Clinical features

The clinical manifestations of iron accumulation include liver disease (ultimately leading to cirrhosis and an increased risk of hepatocellular carcinoma), skin pigmentation, diabetes mellitus, arthropathy, and hypogonadism. Cardiac effects can be the presenting manifestation in 15% of patients, and these include
- Cardiac dysfunction
- Conduction disease.

Investigations

- Routine biochemistry including thyroid and liver function.
- Iron studies (ferritin, transferrin saturation, serum iron, TIBC).
- Genotyping (C282Y homozygosity).
- ECG.
- Echo.

Treatment

Venesection and chelation therapy can be associated with an improvement of ventricular dysfunction. However, irreversible myocardial dysfunction can occur in subjects with advanced disease.

Fig 19.4 (See colour plate 3) Haemochromatosis. Granular intracellular cardiac myocyte deposits of haemosiderin are stained blue. Perls stain ×400. Courtesy of Dr Allan McPhaden, Glasgow Royal Infirmary.

HIV cardiomyopathy

Cardiac involvement occurs in around 50% of patients with the human immunodeficiency virus (HIV), although this is infrequently clinically significant. The exact pathogenesis of HIV cardiomyopathy is not fully established, but thought to include infection of myocardial cells with HIV type 1 (HIV-1), or a subsequent opportunistic infection, and cardiotoxicity from pharmacologic agents (e.g. nucleoside analogues and pentamidine). HIV-1 genomic material has been demonstrated within cardiac myocytes in patients with cardiomyopathy at autopsy.

In a 5-year echocardiographic follow-up study of 952 asymptomatic HIV patients, 8% developed a dilated cardiomyopathy. Of this group:
- The incidence was higher if the CD4 count was <400cells/mm^3.
- A histological diagnosis of myocarditis was made in 83%.
- HIV nucleic acid sequences were found in 76%.
- Inflammatory infiltrates were predominantly composed of CD3 and CD8 lymphocytes.
- In those with active myocarditis, patients were also infected with:
  - Coxsackie B (17%).
  - Cytomegalovirus (6%).
  - Epstein–Barr virus (3%).

⚠ Although this study was published in the *N Engl J Med* (Barbaro G *et al.* Incidence of dilated cardiomyopathy and detection of HIV in myocardial cells of HIV-positive patients. Gruppo Italiano per lo Studio Cardiologico dei Pazienti Affetti da AIDS. *N Engl J Med* 1998; **339**: 1093–9), the work was later retracted by the journal's editors (*N Engl J Med* 2002; **347**: 140) and therefore the validity of the data is uncertain.

Treatment

Conventional HF treatment may help improve cardiac function, even in asymptomatic HIV-positive patients. Caution should be employed when initiating lipid-lowering therapy, due to the interactions between HIV protease inhibitors and statins affecting cytochrome P450 function. Beware also the possible interaction between protease inhibitors and β-adrenoreceptor antagonists, digoxin, or non-dihydropyridine calcium antagonists due to the possible prolongation of AV conduction.

▶ A rare but important differential diagnosis of HIV cardiomyopathy is infective myocarditis (e.g. myocardial toxoplasmosis, aspergillosis, tuberculosis, cryptococcosis, histoplasmosis, candidosis, herpes simplex, cytomegalovirus) or cardiac malignancy.

Chagas' disease

Chagas' disease is a protozoal myocarditis endemic to South and Central America, caused by the parasite *Trypanosoma cruzi*. Between 16 and 18 million people are infected with *T. cruzi* in Latin America. About 70–90% of those infected are asymptomatic carriers and never develop any symptoms.

Acute Chagas' disease tends to be diagnosed most frequently in children, although individuals of all ages can be infected. It can cause a severe myocarditis, particularly in the young, resulting in heart failure and a high risk of mortality. However, if chronic disease occurs, the manifestations are usually delayed and typically do not arise until 20 years later. Whether the features that arise are due directly to parasite invasion or to secondary autoimmune mechanisms is not clear.

Transmission and pathophysiology

The major route of transmission of *T. cruzi* is directly from the reduviid bug. However, the infection can also arise from other routes, including animal reservoirs, blood transfusion, organ transplantation, and vertical transmission. Organs involved show chronic inflammatory changes and diffuse fibrosis due antibody and cell-mediated immunity against *T. cruzi* antigens.

Clinical features

- Fatigue and fluid retention.
- Conduction system disease.
- Progressive cardiac dysfunction.
- Ventricular arrhythmias and sudden death.
- Thrombo-embolic disease.

Investigation

- Machado-Guerreiro complement fixation test.
- Indirect immunofluorescence or ELISA.
- Echo—global LVSD, although in advanced disease there may be posterior hypokinesis with relative sparing of the septal wall. An apical aneurysm may also be a feature.

Treatment

- Anti-parasitic agents (e.g. benznidazole) reduce parasitaemia, but have not been shown to eradicate the disease.
- Standard CHF therapy (not evidence based).
- Anti-arrhythmic drugs (e.g. amiodarone).
- Anticoagulation.

Key reference

Rassi Jr, Rassi A & Little WC. Chagas' heart disease. *Clin Cardiol* 2000; **23**: 883–9.

Lyme disease

Lyme disease is a multi-system disease caused by infection from a tick-borne spirochete (*Borrelia burgdorferi*). Early features include erythema migrans and constitutional upset, but the development of cardiac, neurological, and joint involvement may follow after weeks to months. In the USA, cardiac involvement occurs in up to 10% of untreated adults during the early disseminated phase of the disease—usually within the first two months after infection. This is less common in Europe, possibly related to infection by different organisms. Interestingly, although Lyme disease is seen to have a slight female predominance, the cardiac manifestations are much more common in males (3:1).

Clinical features
- Erythema migrans (approximately 90%).
- Early disseminated features (days to months later).
  - Carditis—the most common manifestation being conduction system disease—often progressing rapidly from first to higher degrees of block over a relatively short period of time, frequently requiring temporary transvenous pacing. Myopericarditis and cardiomyopathy may also develop, but these are generally mild and self-limiting.
  - Neurological—e.g. lymphocytic meningitis, cranial nerve palsies.
  - Migratory polyarthritis (approximately 50%).
- Late features (weeks to years later).
  - Chronic arthritis.
  - Neurological problems, for example, dementia.

Diagnosis and investigation
- History of tick bite, and clinical features of Lyme disease.
- Serological studies with ELISA and western blot to confirm diagnosis.

Treatment

Lyme disease should generally be treated by those experienced in its management. Doxycycline is currently the antibacterial of choice for early Lyme disease, and intravenous ceftriaxone is recommended for Lyme disease associated with moderate to severe cardiac or neurological abnormalities, late Lyme disease, and Lyme arthritis. The duration of treatment is generally 2–4 weeks although Lyme arthritis requires longer treatment with oral antibacterial drugs.

Arrhythmogenic right ventricular cardiomyopathy

Arrhythmogenic right ventricular cardiomyopathy (ARVC) is characterized by the gradual replacement of myocytes by adipose and fibrous tissue primarily in the RV. ARVC is an important cause of sudden death in individuals <30 years (3% SCD/year), and diffuse RV, and occasionally LV, involvement may result in heart failure. The prevalence of ARVC is approximately 1 in 5000.

ARVC is typically inherited as an autosomal dominant trait with variable (approximately 30%) penetrance and incomplete expression. The genes responsible for ARVC have been mapped to chromosomes 1, 2, 3, and 10 and 14. It is understood to be a desmosome disease with defects in desmoplakin, plakoglobulin, and plakophilin. Naxos disease is an autosomal recessive ARVC mapped to chromosome 17, which is characterized by non-epidermolytic palmoplantar keratosis and woolly hair.

Clinical features
ARVC typically occurs in young adult males, and is usually asymptomatic. However, it should be considered in young patients presenting with syncope, VT (usually of RV origin—LBBB morphology), cardiac arrest, or in adult patients with CHF. In the USA, ARVC accounts for approximately 5% of SCD in those <65 years. Heart failure is predominantly right-sided, but may progress to biventricular failure. Most cases are diagnosed before the age of 40.

Investigation and diagnosis
The histological finding of transmural fibrofatty replacement of RV myocardium allows a definitive diagnosis of ARVC. Endomyocardial biopsy has a low sensitivity, since the disease is segmental and rarely involves the interventricular septum. Echocardiography reveals RV dilatation/dysfunction, and cardiac MRI can help to distinguish fat from muscle as well as providing information about RV wall motion and function. An expert consensus group has proposed the criteria for the diagnosis (see opposite).

Treatment
β-adrenoreceptor antagonists are first-line therapy (± amiodarone) for those with well-tolerated ventricular arrhythmias and for those with LVSD. Verapamil is an alternative in those that who intolerant to this regime but caution should be employed in CHF. Radiofrequency ablation can be considered in patients who are unresponsive/intolerant to antiarrhythmic drugs, although this has a limited success rate due to the diffuse and progressive nature of the disease. Patients who are considered to be at high risk for sudden cardiac death should receive an ICD.

Criteria for diagnosis of ARVC—a patient must demonstrate either two major criteria, one major criteria plus two minor criteria, or four minor criteria.

1. Global or regional dysfunction and structural alterations[*]

Major:
- Severe dilation and reduction of RV ejection fraction with no (or only mild) LV impairment.
- Localized RV aneurysms.
- Severe segmental dilation of the RV.

Minor:
- Mild global RV dilation or ejection fraction reduction with normal LV.
- Mild segmental dilation of the RV.
- Regional RV hypokinesia.

2. Tissue characterization of walls

Major:
- Fibrofatty replacement of myocardium on endomyocardial biopsy.

3. Repolarization abnormalities

Minor:
- Inverted T waves in right pre-cordial leads (V_2 and V_3) (people aged >12 years; in the absence of right bundle branch block).

4. Depolarization/conduction abnormalities

Major:
- Epsilon waves or localized prolongation (>110ms) of the QRS complex in right pre-cordial leads (V_1 to V_3).

Minor:
- Late potentials (signal-averaged ECG).

5. Arrhythmia

Minor:
- Ventricular tachycardia of LBBB morphology.
- Frequent ventricular extrasystoles (>1000/24 hours on Holter).

6. Family history

Major:
- Familial disease confirmed at necropsy or surgery.

Minor:
- Familial history of premature sudden death (<35 years) due to suspected RV cardiomyopathy.
- Familial history (clinical diagnosis based on the present criteria).

[*] Echo, angiography, magnetic resonance imaging, or radionuclide scintigraphy

Key reference

Reproduced from McKenna WJ et al. Diagnosis of arrhythmogenic right ventricular dysplasia/cardiomyopathy. Task Force of the Working Group Myocardial and Pericardial Disease of the European Society of Cardiology and of the Scientific Council on Cardiomyopathies of the International Society and Federation of Cardiology. Br Heart J 1994; **71**: 215–8.

Additional key reference: Gemayel C, Pelliccia A & Thompson PD Arrhythmogenic right ventricular cardiomyopathy. J Am Coll Cardiol 2001; **38**: 1773–81.

Left ventricular non-compaction

Left ventricular non-compaction (LVNC) is an 'unclassified cardiomyopathy' characterized by marked prominent trabeculation and deep intertrabecular recesses within the left ventricle. These alterations are thought to be due to an intrauterine arrest of compaction of the myocardial fibers in the absence of any coexisting congenital lesions.

There is a familial link with around half of the patients having affected family members. The pattern of inheritance is generally autosomal dominant, although cases with X-linked inheritance have been recognized. Several mutations have been described, including genes coding for the proteins α-dystrobrevin, tafazzin, Cypher/ZASP, and lamin A/C.

Clinical features

LVNC can be either isolated or non-isolated. The latter form may be found in combination with septal defects, pulmonary stenosis, or hypoplastic left ventricle. LVNC can be associated with a high incidence of heart failure, thromboembolism, and ventricular arrhythmias.

Mortality and morbidity rates are variable, but are high in those who have symptoms of severe CHF, sustained ventricular arrhythmias, or left atrial enlargement.

Investigation

The diagnosis can be made by echocardiography or MRI with appearances of a non-compacted sub-endocardial layer of trabecularization with deep endomyocardial recesses. This most commonly involves the lateral, apical, and inferior walls of the left ventricle.

Treatment

- Standard CHF therapy.
- Anti-coagulation due to risk of thromboembolism.
- Family screening.

Key reference

Lofiego C et al. Wide spectrum of presentation and variable outcomes of isolated left ventricular non-compaction. *Heart* 2007; **93**: 65–71.

Hypertrophic cardiomyopathy

Hypertrophic cardiomyopathy (HCM) is a common genetic disorder characterized by the presence of unexplained left ventricular hypertrophy. This classically causes asymmetric hypertrophy of the interventricular septum (IVS), but there is significant heterogeneity in the extent of cardiac hypertrophy and degree of outflow obstruction, the latter of which is thought to affect 25% of individuals. By the time patients with HCM present with HF, the morphology may have changed from hypertrophic to dilated cardiomyopathy.

Aetiology

HCM has an autosomal dominant inheritance, with incomplete penetrance. Several genes have been associated with HCM, each of them encoding cardiac sarcomere proteins (see Table 19.1 and Table 19.2, p. 253). Histologically, HCM has the distinctive appearance of myocyte disarray—where hypertrophied cardiomyocytes form abnormal intercellular connections—and fibrosis. The incidence is approximately 1:500.

Clinical features

Many affected individuals are asymptomatic and are picked up incidentally. However, the first clinical manifestation may be sudden death, and therefore there is a significant variability in clinical course as well as outcome. Symptoms may include:

- Breathlessness—impaired ventricular filling (↑ LVEDP).
- Fatigue.
- Chest pain.
- Arrhythmias—both atrial and ventricular.
- Syncope.

Examination may be normal, although signs include:

- Jerky pulse.
- Prominent a-wave in JVP.
- Laterally displaced ± double apex beat.
- S_4.
- Harsh systolic murmur at left sternal edge, increasing with Valsalva maneuver, or on standing from a squat position.

Investigations

- ECG—usually abnormal (85%), with ST/T wave abnormalities and LVH particularly in the mid-pre-cordial leads. Prominent inferior or pre-cordial Q-waves are also frequently seen (in up to 50%).
- Echocardiography:
  - Degree and distribution of ventricular hypertrophy.
  - Small cavity size.
  - Outflow tract obstruction (caused by a thickened IVS and systolic anterior motion of the anterior mitral valve leaflet (SAM)).
  - Normal systolic function (although LVSD occurs in 5–10%).

Table 19.2 Causes of left ventricular hypertrophy

Sarcomeric protein disease
- β-myosin heavy chain.
- Cardiac myosin binding protein C.
- Cardiac troponin I.
- Troponin-T.
- α-Tropomyosin.
- Essential myosin light chain.
- Regulatory myosin light chain.
- Cardiac α-actin.
- α-myosin heavy chain.
- Titin.
- Troponin C.

Metabolic disease
- Glycogen storage disease II) Pompe's disease.
- (Glycogen storage disease III) Forbes' disease.
- Anderson-Fabry disease.
- Carnitine deficiency.
- Phosphorylase B Kinase deficiency.
- Infant of diabetic mother.
- AMP Kinase (WPW, HCM, conduction disease).
- Debrancher enzyme deficiency.
- Hurler's syndrome.
- Hurler–Scheie disease.
- Hunter's syndrome.
- Mannosidosis.
- Fucosidosis.
- Total lipodystrophy.
- Mitochondrial cytopathy.
  - MELAS.
  - MERRF.
  - LHON.

Syndromic HCM
- Noonan's syndrome.
- LEOPARD syndrome.
- Friedreich's ataxia.
- Beckwith–Wiedermann syndrome.
- Swyer's syndrome (pure gonadal dysgenesis).

Miscellaneous
- Obesity.
- Athletic training.
- Muscle LIM protein.
- Phospholamban promoter.
- Amyloidosis.
- Phaeochromocytoma.

WPW = Wolff–Parkinson–White syndrome. HCM = hypertrophic cardiomyopathy.
MELAS = mitochondrial encephalomyopathy, lactic acidosis, and stroke-like episodes.
MERRF = myoclonic epilepsy and ragged red fibres. LHON = Leber's hereditary optic neuropathy.

Reproduced from: Elliott P & McKenna WJ. *Lancet* 2004; **363**: 1881–91 with permission from Elsevier

Other investigations

- Cardiac MRI.
- Ambulatory ECG recording—to assess for arrhythmias.
- Exercise testing—to assess functional capacity and BP response.
- Genetic testing.

Treatment

Pharmacological

- β-adrenoreceptor antagonists are the cornerstone of HCM therapy. By reducing heart rate, they reduce myocardial oxygen demand (and thus symptoms of angina and breathlessness), and an increase in out-flow tract obstruction that accompanies exercise. β-adrenoreceptor antagonists are also anti-arrhythmic agents and may reduce the risk of syncope and SCD. Caution should be employed in the withdrawal of these agents due to rebound sympathetic sensitivity.
- Calcium channel antagonists (particularly verapamil) can be used in patients intolerant to β-adrenoreceptor antagonists.
- Anti-arrhythmic agents—amiodarone is an effective anti-arrhythmic agent, but has not been shown to conclusively reduce the risk of SCD. Disopyramide can reduce the outflow gradient and may lead to symptomatic improvement, although these benefits may diminish with time.

Non-pharmacological

- Surgical myotomy–myectomy (Morrow procedure)—transaortic resection of IVS to debulk the septum. This is associated with a ~1% mortality and 5% risk of complete heart block (CHB). It may be combined with a mitral valve replacement in patients with significant SAM of the mitral valve.
- Alcohol septal ablation is considered in those patients felt unsuitable for surgical myotomy–myectomy. It is performed by inducing a localized septal infarction. Alcohol is injected into the first or second septal perforator artery, following a contrast injection to ensure the correct septal distribution. The risk of CHB is approximately 15%.
- Dual chamber pacing should be considered in symptomatic individuals with an outflow tract gradient, who are not felt suitable for surgical myectomy or alcohol septal ablation. By programming a short a-v delay, the outflow gradient can be reduced by 50%.
- ICD—should be considered in high-risk individuals (see opposite), particularly those with sustained ventricular arrhythmias and following resuscitated cardiac arrest. In the presence of outflow obstruction, a dual chamber ICD is potentially of value (see dual chamber pacing above).

Exercise

Undiagnosed HCM is the most common autopsy finding in competitive athletes who die suddenly. It is also true that around 50% of HCM deaths occur with or following exercise; therefore, strenuous activity should be avoided.

Risk factors in HCM

- History of SCD.
- Family history of premature death.
- History of syncope.
- Magnitude of left ventricular hypertrophy (>30mm).
- Abnormal blood pressure response to exercise.
- Presence of non-sustained VT on Holter.
- LV outflow tract obstruction (>30mmHg at rest).
- Early onset of the disease.
- Myocardial ischemia on perfusion tomography.
- 'Malignant' causal mutations.
- 'Malignant' modifier genes.
- Extent of myocyte disarray.
- Extent of interstitial fibrosis.

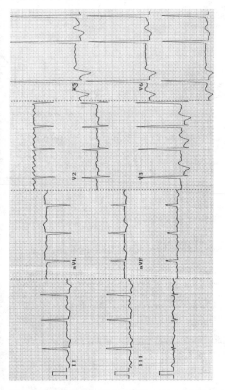

Fig. 19.5 ECG of HCM. Reproduced from Myerson SG et al. (2005) *Emergencies in Cardiology*, p. 81 with permission from Oxford University Press.

Restrictive cardiomyopathy

Restrictive cardiomyopathy is an uncommon condition in Western countries, characterized by impaired diastolic function secondary to reduced ventricular compliance. In certain geographical locations (particularly the tropics—Africa, India, South and Central America, and Asia), restrictive cardiomyopathy is a more important cause of death due to the higher incidence of endomyocardial fibrosis in those regions. Systolic function usually remains normal, at least early in the disease.

Aetiology

Although the aetiology is often obscure, there are several known causes of restrictive cardiomyopathy:

- Endomyocardial.
  - Endomyocardial fibrosis.
  - Hypereosinophilic syndrome (Löffler endocarditis).
  - Carcinoid and metastatic disease.
  - Radiation.
  - Anthracycline therapy.
- Myocardial.
  - Infiltrative (e.g. amyloid, sarcoid, Gaucher disease).
  - Non-infiltrative (e.g. scleroderma).
  - Storage diseases (e.g. haemochromatosis, glycogen and lysosomal storage disease).

Clinical features

- Exercise intolerance (limited increase in cardiac output secondary to fixed stroke volume).
- Elevated filling pressures.
- Impalpable apex beat (unlike constrictive pericarditis).
- S_3/S_4.
- Peripheral oedema.
- Hepatomegaly and ascites.
- Kussmaul sign (inspiratory increase in JVP).

Investigations

- ECG—P mitrale/pulmonale; low pre-cordial QRS amplitude; atrial arrhythmias.
- Echocardiography—may initially appear unremarkable, with normal ventricular dimensions and systolic function. However, there is often marked bi-atrial enlargement secondary to elevated atrial pressures, and a restrictive inflow pattern seen on mitral Doppler.
- Cardiac catheterization to differentiate from constrictive pericarditis (see Table 19.3).
- CT/MRI—assessment for infiltrative myocardial and endomyocardial disease, as well as imaging of the pericardium.

Treatment

- Diuretic therapy for fluid overload.
- Avoidance of or rate control in AF will help maintain ventricular filling time.
- Specific therapy directed towards underlying cause.

▶ Beware of underfilling patients with restrictive cardiomyopathy, as a drop in filling pressure will have a marked impact on cardiac output).

▶ Differentiation from constrictive pericarditis is important as this can be treated surgically by pericardectomy (see Table 19.3).

Prognosis

The prognosis of restrictive cardiomyopathy is generally poor.

Table 19.3 Features differentiating constrictive pericarditis from restrictive cardiomyopathy

Feature	Constrictive pericarditis	Restrictive cardiomyopathy
Past medical history	Previous pericarditis, cardiac surgery, trauma, radiotherapy, connective tissue disease	These items rare
Jugular venous waveform	X and Y dips brief and 'flicking', not conspicuous positive waves	X and Y dips less brief, may have conspicuous A wave or V wave
Extra sounds in diastole	Early S_3, high pitched 'pericardial knock'. No S_4	Later S_3, low pitched, 'triple rhythm', S_4 in some cases
Mitral or tricuspid regurgitation	Usually absent	Often present
ECG	P waves reflect intra-atrial conduction delay. Atrioventricular or intraventricular conduction defects rare	P waves reflect right or left atrial hypertrophy or overload. Atrioventricular or intraventricular' conduction defects not unusual
Plain chest radiograph	Pericardial calcification in 20–30%	Pericardial calcification rare
Ventricular septal movement in diastole	Abrupt septal movement ('notch') in early diastole in most cases	Abrupt septal movement in early diastole seen only occasionally
Ventricular septal movement with respiration	Notable movement towards left ventricle in inspiration usually seen	Relatively little movement towards left ventricle in most cases
Atrial enlargement	Slight or moderate in most cases	Pronounced in most cases

Respiratory variation in mitral and tricuspid flow velocity	>25% in most cases	<15% in most cases
Equilibration of diastolic pressures in all cardiac chambers	Within 5mmHg in nearly all cases, often essentially the same	Within 5mmHg in a small proportion of cases
Dip–plateau waveform in the right ventricular pressure waveform	End diastolic pressure more than one-third of systolic pressure in many cases	End diastolic pressure often less than one-third of systolic
Peak right ventricular systolic pressure	Nearly always <60mmHg, often <40mmHg	Frequently >40mmHg and occasionally >60mmHg
Discordant respiratory variation of ventricular peak systolic pressures	Right and left ventricular peak systolic pressure variations are out-of-phase	Right and left ventricular peak systolic pressure variations are in-phase
Paradoxical pulse	Often present to a moderate degree	Rarely present
MR/CT imaging	Shows thick pericardium in most cases	Shows thick pericardium only rarely
Endomyocardial biopsy	Normal, or non-specific abnormalities	Shows amyloid in some cases, rarely other specific infiltrative disease

Reproduced from Hancock EW. Differential diagnosis of restrictive cardiomyopathy and constrictive pericarditis. *Heart* 2001; **86**: 343–9 (table 3) with permission from BMJ Publishing Group Ltd.

Cardiac amyloidosis

Cardiac amyloidosis is an uncommon, but likely underdiagnosed, condition. There are several types of amyloid, each with its unique features and treatment. The common feature of this group of diseases is the extracellular deposition of proteinaceous matter, which demonstrates apple-green birefringence under polarized light when stained with Congo red (Figs. 19.6 and 19.7).

Cardiac amyloid deposits result in:
• Biventricular wall thickening, but not dilatation.
• Restrictive type cardiomyopathy.
• Systolic dysfunction in advanced disease.
• Atrial dilatation.
• Valvular involvement.
• Conduction system involvement.
• Perivascular involvement (particularly small vessels).

AL amyloidosis

AL amyloid is the commonest form of amyloidosis. It is associated with a plasma cell dyscrasia (e.g. multiple myeloma), with the amyloid produced from clonal light chains. Cardiac involvement is in around half of the patients with AL amyloidosis, and its presence identifies a high-risk individual. Few patients have isolated cardiac involvement only.

Clinical features
• Rapidly progressive signs and symptoms—median survival = 15 months.
• Periorbital purpura (virtually pathognomonic) and easy bruising
• Macroglossia (10–20%).
• Carpal tunnel syndrome.
• Progressive dyspnoea is common, almost always associated with evidence of elevated right-sided filling pressure.
• Marked peripheral oedema and ascites.
• Weight loss.
• Chest pain due to amyloid deposition in the small vessels of the heart.
• Sudden death is common, but not due to ventricular arrhythmias.
• Atrial arrhythmias (particularly AF) occur in 15%, and are associated with a very high incidence of thromboembolism.
• Hypotension/postural hypotension.
• Hepatomegaly.
• Autonomic/sensory neuropathy.
• Nephrotic syndrome.

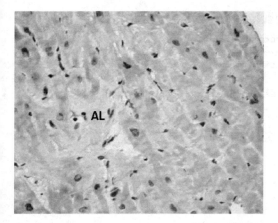

Fig 19.6 (See colour plate 4) Histopathology of cardiac amyloid, demonstrating apple green birefringence with polarized light. Courtesy of Dr Allan McPhaden, Glasgow Royal Infirmary.

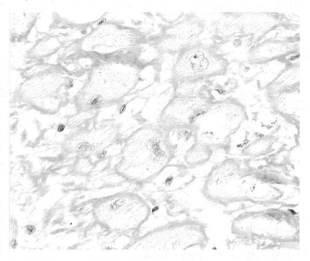

Fig 19.7 (See colour plate 5) Amyloidosis—Individual myocytes are ringed by pink-staining extracellullar deposits of amyloid in a case of primary amyloidosis. Sirius red ×400. Courtesy of Dr Allan McPhaden, Glasgow Royal Infirmary.

Investigation of AL amyloidosis

Electrocardiographic features

- Abnormal axis.
- Reduced voltage out of keeping with ventricular thickness.
- Bundle branch block is unusual (particularly LBBB), unless pre-existing.

Echocardiographic features (Fig. 19.8)

- Non-dilated ventricles.
- Concentric biventricular thickening.
- Essentially normal ejection fraction until advanced disease.
- Granular infiltration of the atrial and ventricular septum.
- Restrictive Doppler pattern in advanced disease.
- Tissue Doppler and strain rate imaging may have a role.

Cardiac magnetic resonance

- Global sub-endocardial late gadolinium enhancement.
- Abnormal myocardial and blood-pool gadolinium kinetics.

Cardiac catheterization

- Elevated left ventricular end-diastolic pressure (LVEDP).
- Dip-and-plateau waveform on pressure tracings.
- LVEDP exceeds right ventricular end-diastolic pressure by >7mmHg.

Tissue diagnosis

- Fine-needle aspiration of the abdominal fat is positive for amyloid deposits in >70% of patients with AL amyloidosis.
- Apple-green birefringence when stained with Congo red and viewed under polarized light.
- Endomyocardial biopsy is virtually 100% sensitive, because AL amyloid is widely deposited throughout the heart.

Other investigations

- Search for the presence of a plasma cell dyscrasia (most to least sensitive).
  - Serum free-light-chain assay.
  - Serum and urine immunofixation.
  - Urine electrophoresis.
- Bone marrow biopsy.

In AL amyloidosis, free lambda or (less commonly) free kappa levels are elevated.

Management

Treatment of the underlying disease

- Antiplasma cell therapy (e.g. melphalan)
- AL amyloidosis is generally seen as a contra-indication to cardiac transplantation.

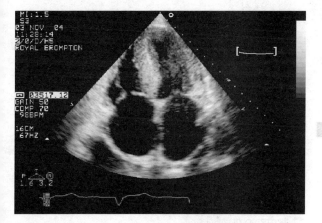

Fig. 19.8 Restrictive cardiomyopathy secondary to amyloid infiltration, with classical septal granular thickening and biatrial enlargement.

Treatment of cardiac-related symptoms in AL amyloidosis
- Diuretics—the mainstay of heart failure therapy due to amyloidosis. High doses may be needed in coexisting nephrotic syndrome.
- ACE inhibitors and ARBs are very poorly tolerated due to hypotension.
- β-Blockers are of unknown safety and efficacy.
- Anticoagulation should be strongly considered in patients with atrial fibrillation due to the very high rate of thrombo-embolic events.

⚠ Digoxin—increased risk of digoxin toxicity because the drug binds avidly to amyloid fibrils, even with therapeutic serum digoxin levels.

Secondary amyloidosis
Cardiac amyloid deposition in secondary amyloidosis is very rare, and hepatic and renal amyloid deposition dominates the clinical picture. It is associated with:
- Chronic infections.
- Rheumatoid arthritis.
- Other rheumatic disorders such as ankylosing spondylitis.
- Inflammatory bowel disease.

Isolated atrial amyloidosis
Isolated atrial amyloidosis is a common finding at autopsy, particularly in elderly patients, and involvement is strictly limited to the atria. It originates from atrial natriuretic peptide, and its significance is currently uncertain. However, it is more likely to be found in patients with atrial fibrillation.

Hereditary amyloidosis
Hereditary amyloidosis is a heterogenous condition with most cases due to an altered transthyretin protein. It is autosomal dominant with high penetrance. The definitive treatment is liver transplantation, which removes the source of transthyretin and thus the precursor of amyloid deposition. There are other, very rare, causes of familial non-transthyretin amyloidosis, but amyloid deposition is predominantly in organs other than the heart.

Senile cardiac amyloidosis (SCA)
SCA is the clinical manifestation of senile systemic amyloidosis. It results from the cardiac deposition of amyloid derived from wild-type transthyretin, and is almost exclusively found in men over 70 years of age. The median survival from the onset of heart failure is 7 years, and the condition invariably presents as congestive heart failure. The echocardiographic appearance is identical to that found in patients with AL amyloidosis; and as non-cardiac involvement is rare, the diagnosis is confirmed by endomyocardial biopsy. Bifascicular and complete heart block are common, often necessitating permanent pacemaker implantation. Atrial fibrillation is also common and, like in AL amyloid, anticoagulation is advised.

Endomyocardial disease

Endomyocardial fibrosis (EMF) is characterized by fibrous endocardial involvement of either/both ventricles, often with associated atrioventricular valvular regurgitation. EMF typically occurs in equatorial Africa, where it is a frequent cause of chronic heart failure. It is also recognized elsewhere: generally within 15° of the equator.

Clinical features and investigation

- LV (40%), RV (10%), or biventricular involvement (50%).
- Subsequent atrial enlargement.
- MR/TR.
- Symptoms and signs of left/right ventricular failure.
- Pericardial effusion—may be large.
- Eosinophilia may be present.
- Mural thrombi common.
- ECG—small QRS voltages; ST/T wave abnormalities.
- Echo—apical obliteration of involved ventricle; dilated atria, pericardial effusion; MR/TR.
- Endomyocardial biopsy may be diagnostic.

Treatment

- Diuretics.
- Anticoagulation.
- AF can be rate-controlled with digoxin, but its occurrence heralds a poor prognosis.
- Surgical removal of fibrotic endocardium leads to a significant improvement in symptoms, although recurrent fibrosis invariably occurs.

Löffler endocarditis (the hypereosinophilic syndrome)

Hypereosinophilic syndrome (HES) is a clinical diagnosis where there is a sustained eosinophil count >1500/mm^3 for 6 months, with organ involvement. Most patients with HES have biventricular cardiac involvement (Löffler endocarditis), with eosinophilic myocarditis, mural thrombosis, and fibrotic change, resulting in a restrictive cardiomyopathy.

Clinical features and investigations

- Systemic upset—fever, weight loss, rash, cough.
- Symptoms and signs of heart failure.
- Atrial fibrillation is common.
- Thromboembolic disease.
- Associated involvement of the lungs, bone marrow, brain, and kidneys.
- ECG—non-specific T wave abnormalities.
- Echo—localized thickening of the LV basal posterior wall; restricted motion of the posterior mitral valve leaflet; preserved systolic function; dilated atria, apical thrombus.

Treatment
- Diuretics and vasodilators.
- Anticoagulation.
- Corticosteroids ± hydroxyurea.
- Interferon may be tried in advanced cases.
- Surgical removal of fibrotic endocardium.

Myocarditis

Myocarditis is the inflammation of myocardium due to one of a large number of causes (see following sections), including infection (either acute or as a post-infectious autoimmune response), systemic disease, drugs, and toxins. Currently, the most frequently implicated virus in developed countries is parvovirus B19, although other viruses are commonly implicated.

Myocardial inflammation may be focal or diffuse, involving any or all cardiac chambers. The clinical course is variable—from full recovery to sudden death or the need for urgent cardiac transplantation. This variability appears, in part, to be due to the underlying aetiology.

Classification[1]

- **Fulminant**—preceding flu-like illness, with a distinct onset of cardiac symptoms and rapid deterioration. Patients present with shock or symptoms or signs of severe LVSD. The clinical course is variable and patients either recover over the space of a few weeks or deteriorate rapidly requiring consideration of CTx. Endomyocardial biopsy shows active myocarditis. Immunosuppressive therapy is ineffective.
- **Acute**— unclear onset with gradual decline in cardiac function. Patients present with symptoms of progressive HF and ventricular dilatation with LVSD. There is active or borderline myocarditis on biopsy, which resolves with time. Patients either respond to CHF therapy or progress to dilated cardiomyopathy.
- **Chronic active**— onset indistinct with progressive deterioration, present with CHF with LVSD. Initial biopsy shows active or borderline myocarditis; however, subsequent biopsy reveals continued inflammation, fibrosis, giant cells, with eventual development of a dilated cardiompyopathy
- **Chronic persistent**—no distinct onset of symptoms (primarily chest pain or palpitations) characterized by a persistent infiltrate on biopsy, often with foci of myocyte necrosis but without ventricular dysfunction. Immunosuppressive therapy does not affect myocardial infiltrate or clinical outcome.

Causes of myocarditis[2]

Infectious

- *Viral*—Adenovirus, Arbovirus (dengue fever, yellow fever), Arenavirus (lassa fever), Coxsackie virus, Cytomegalovirus, Echovirus, Encephalomyocarditis virus, Epstein–Barr virus, Hepatitis B, Herpesvirus, HIV-1, Influenza virus, Mumps virus, Poliomyelitis virus, Rabies, Respiratory Syncytial virus, Rubella virus, Rubeola virus, Vaccinia virus, Varicella virus, Variola virus (Fig. 19.9).
- *Bacterial*—Brucellosis, Clostridia, Diphtheria, Franciella, Gonococcus, Haemophilus, Legionella, Meningococcus, Mycobacteria, Mycoplasma, Pneumococcus, Psittacosis, Salmonella, Staphylococcus, Streptococcus, *Tropheryma whippelii* (Whipple's disease)
- *Fungal*—Actinomyces, Aspergillus, Blastomyces, Candida, Coccidioides, Cryptococcus, Histoplasma, Nocardia, Sporothrix

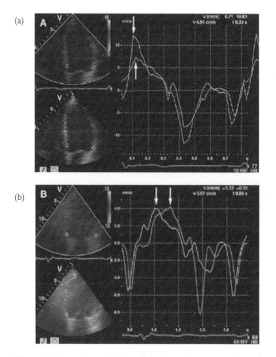

Plate 1 (Also see Fig. 6.1) Colour-coded tissue Doppler images, four-chamber views. Left ventricular dyssynchrony is defined as the delay in peak systolic velocities between the basal septum and the basal lateral wall.

(a). Tracings from a normal individual. The arrows indicate the peak systolic velocities, illustrating perfect synchrony between the two walls.

(b). Tracings showing extensive left-ventricular dyssynchrony in a patient with severe heart failure. The arrows indicate the peak systolic velocity in each curve, illustrating dyssynchrony of 130ms duration. The tissue Doppler tracings are obtained from samples placed in the basal part of the septum (yellow curve) and the lateral wall (green curve).

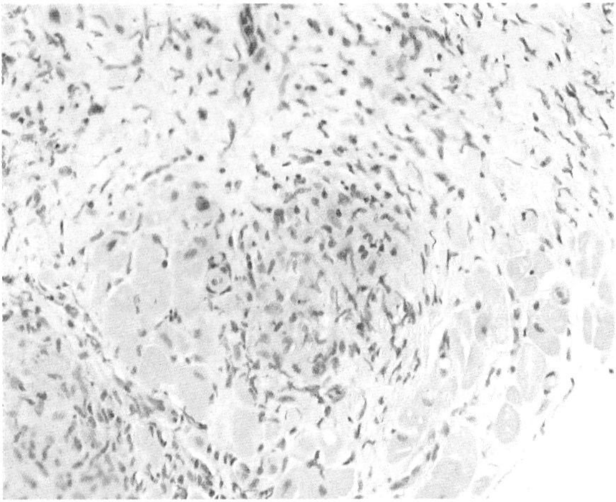

Plate 2 (Also see Fig. 19.3) Sarcoidosis. A central non-caseating granuloma is disrupting the myocardium with myocyte destruction and early replacement fibrosis. A second granuloma is present at the bottom left. Haematoxylin and eosin ×400.

Plate 3 (Also see Fig. 19.4) Haemochromatosis. Granular intracellular cardiac myocyte deposits of haemosiderin are stained blue. Perls stain ×400.

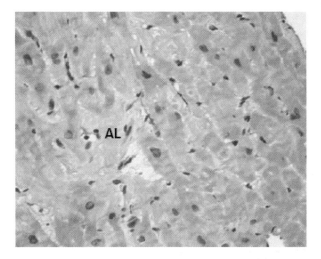

Plate 4 (Also see Fig. 19.6) Histopathology of cardiac amyloid, demonstrating apple green birefringence with polarized light.

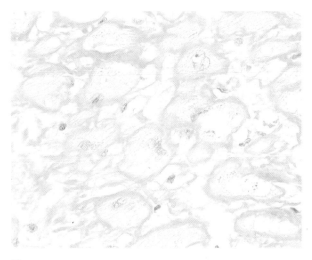

Plate 5 (Also see Fig. 19.7) Amyloidosis—Individual myocytes are ringed by pink-staining extracellullar deposits of amyloid in a case of primary amyloidosis. Sirius red ×400.

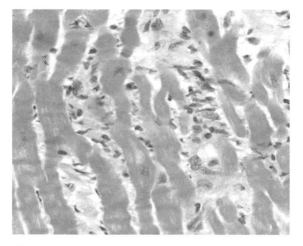

Plate 6 (Also see Fig. 19.9) Viral myocarditis. The myocardium contains focal interstitial infiltration by mononuclear cells, with associated cardiac myocyte degeneration. Haematoxylin and eosin x400.

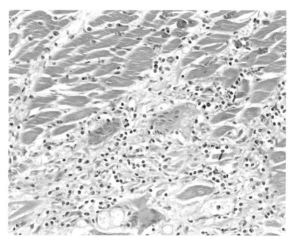

Plate 7 (Also see Fig. 19.10) Giant cell myocarditis. The myocardium is being damaged by a marked chronic inflammatory infiltrate that includes prominent multi-nucleated giant cells in the bottom half of the image. Haematoxlin and eosin x200.

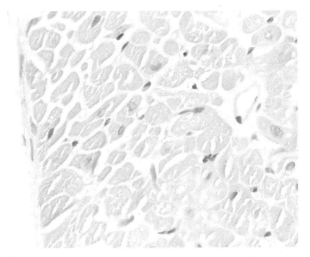

Plate 8 (Also see Fig. 27.1) Normal endocardium and myocardium. The endocardium on the left is a thin uniform layer with underlying myocardium that comprises cardiac myocytes, which are closely applied to one another with little intervening stroma that includes small blood vessels. Haematoxylin and eosin ×400.

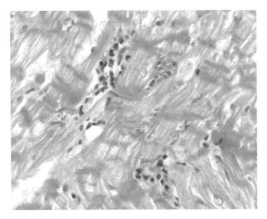

Plate 9 (Also see Fig. 27.2) Low-grade cardiac allograft rejection. The myocardium contains small perivascular aggregates of mononuclear cells (ISHT Grade 1a). Haematoxylin and eosin ×400.

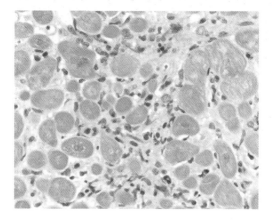

Plate 10 (Also see Fig. 27.3) High-grade cardiac allograft rejection. The myocardium contains perivascular aggregates of mononuclear cells with extension into the interstitium associated with mutiple foci of cardiac myocyte degeneration. Haematoxylin and eosin ×400.

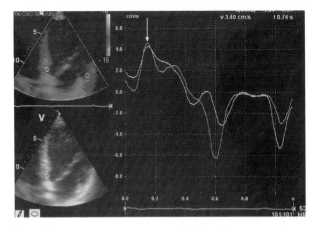

Plate 11 (Also see Fig. 30.1) The assessment of LV dyssynchrony in a normal individual. In the colour-coded tissue Doppler images, sample volumes are placed in the basal part of the septum and lateral wall. Velocity graphs derived from the velocities measured in these sample volumes are presented. LV dyssynchrony is not present, as indicated by a septal-to-lateral delay in peak systolic velocity (↓) of 0ms.

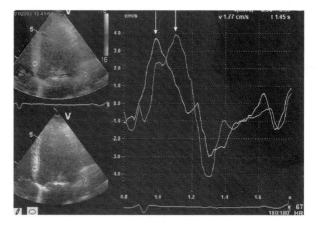

Plate 12 (Also see Fig. 30.2) LV dyssynchrony assessment in CHF. There is extensive LV dyssynchrony with a septal-to-lateral delay in peak systolic velocities of 115ms (the time between the arrows).

- *Rickettsial*—Rocky Mountain spotted fever, Q fever, Scrub Typhus, Typhus
- *Spirochetal*—Borrelia (Lyme's disease), Leptospira, Syphilis
- *Helminthic*—Cysticercus, Echinococcus, Schistosoma, Toxocara (Visceral larva migrans), Trichinella
- *Protozoal*—Entamoeba, Leishmania, Trypanosoma (Chagas's disease), Toxoplasmosis

Non-infectious

- Drug Induced
  - Toxic myocarditis—Amphetamines, Anthracyclines[*], Catecholamines, Chloroquine, Cocaine[*], Cyclophosphamide[*], Emetine, 5-Flouracil, α-Interferon, Interleukin-2[*], Lithium, Paracetamol, Thyroid hormone
  - Hypersensitivity myocarditis—Acetazolamide, Allopurinol, Amitriptyline, Amphotericin B, Ampicillin[*], Carbamazepine, Cephalothin, Chlorthalidone, Colchicine, Diclofenac, Diphenhydramine, Furosemide, Hydrochlorothiazide[*], Indomethacin, Isoniazid, Lidocaine, Methyldopa[*], Methysergide, Oxphenbutazone, Para-aminosalicyclic acid, Penicillins[*], Phenindione, Phenylbutazone, Phenytoin, Procainamide, Pyribenzamine, Reserpine, Spironolactone, Streptomycin, Sulfadiazine[*], Sulfamethoxizole[*], Sulfisoxazole[*], Sulfonylureas, Tetracycline, Trimethaprim
- *Toxins*— Arsenic, Carbon monoxide, Copper, Iron, Lead, Mercury, Phosphorus, Scorpion stings, Snake venom, Spider bites, Wasp sting
- *Systemic diseases*—Arteritis (Giant cell, Takayasau), β-thalassaemia major, Churg-Strauss vasculitis, Crohn's disease, Cryoglobulinemia, Dermatomyositis, Diabetes mellitus, Hashimoto's thyroiditis, Kawasaki's disease[*], Mixed connective tissue disorder, Myesthenia gravis, Periarteritis nodosa, Pernicious anaemia, Pheochromocytoma, Polymyositis, Rheumatoid arthritis, Sarcoidosis[*], Scleroderma, Sjogren's syndrome, Systemic lupus erythematosis[*], Thymoma, Ulcerative colitis, Wegener's granulomatosis
- *Other*— Cardiac rejection[*], Eosinophilic myocarditis, Genetic, Giant cell myocarditis[*], Granulomatous myocarditis, Head Trauma, Hypothermia, Hyperpyrexia, Ionizing radiation, Mononuclear myocarditis, Peripartum myocarditis[*]

[*] More common aetiologies.

Key references

1. Adapted from Lieberman EB et al. Clinicopathologic description of myocarditis. *J Am Coll Cardiol* 1991; **18**: 1617–26.
2. Adapted from Pisani B, Taylor DO & Mason JW. Inflammatory myocardial diseases and cardiomyopathies. *Am J Med* 1997; **102**: 459–69 with permission from Elsevier.

Clinical features

Myocarditis has a variable clinical course, but symptoms and signs include:
- May be asymptomatic.
- Prodromal viral illness—fever, myalgia, fatigue.
- Decreased exercise tolerance.
- Breathlessness.
- Chest pain (particularly in myopericarditis. However, myocarditis can mimic myocardial ischaemia, and therefore should be considered in patients with an acute coronary syndrome and normal coronary arteries).
- Raised JVP.
- S_3/S_4.
- MR/TR.
- Pericardial friction rub (in myopericarditis).
- Peripheral and pulmonary oedema.
- Cardiogenic shock.
- Ventricular arrhythmias and sudden death.

Investigation and diagnosis

- Cardiac troponin—raised concentrations indicate recent onset or ongoing myocardial necrosis.
- WCC/CRP—usually elevated.
- ECG—non-specifically abnormal: ST/T abnormalities, arrhythmias.
- CXR—may be normal; cardiomegaly ± pulmonary oedema.
- ECHO—global, but variable degrees of cardiac dysfunction, MR, TR.
- MRI—may be useful in myocardial characterization, particularly with the use of gadolinium (Gd)-DTPA contrast-enhancement.
- Gallium scanning—may demonstrate myocardial cellular infiltration.
- PCR for the detection of the viral genome in selected cases, although false positive tests do occur.
- Endomyocardial biopsy—may reveal a lymphocytic infiltrate ± myocardial necrosis. The sensitivity may be as low as 35% due to transient and patchy myocardial involvement. The Dallas histopathological criteria were devised in 1986:
  - **Active myocarditis**—'an inflammatory infiltrate of the myocardium with necrosis and/or degeneration of adjacent myocytes not typical of the ischemic damage associated with coronary heart disease'. The infiltrates are usually mononuclear, but may be neutrophilic or, occasionally, eosinophilic.
  - **Borderline myocarditis** is the term used when the inflammatory infiltrate is too sparse, or myocyte injury is not demonstrated, and a repeat biopsy may be indicated.

Treatment

- Bed rest.
- Usual HF therapy—diuretics, ACE inhibitors, β-adrenoreceptor antagonists when euvolaemic.
- Supportive therapy for cardiogenic shock—IABP, inotropes, consideration of VADs/urgent CTx.
- There is no evidence of benefit from immunosuppressive therapy.

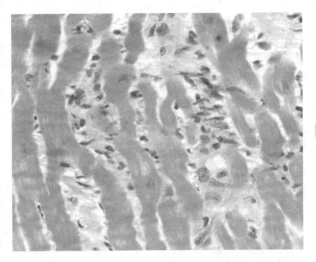

Fig. 19.9 (See colour plate 6) Viral myocarditis. The myocardium contains focal intertstitial infiltration by mononuclear cells, with associated cardiac myocyte degeneration. Haematoxylin and eosin x400. Courtesy of Dr Allan McPhaden, Glasgow Royal Infirmary.

Giant cell myocarditis

Giant cell myocarditis is a rare form of myocarditis that presents with rapidly deteriorating cardiac dysfunction and arrhythmias. Approximately 20% of patients have coexisting autoimmune disease, and the great majority of affected individuals (approximately 90%) are caucasian. Endomyocardial biopsies reveal widespread necrosis and inflammation with the presence of lymphocytes, histiocytes, eosinophils, as well as the characteristic multi-nucleated giant cells (Fig. 19.10).

The prognosis of giant cell myocarditis is very poor (<6 months), and identifying such patients early will allow the immediate administration of multi-drug immunosuppressive therapy (a combination of prednisolone, cyclosporine, azathioprine, or OKT$_3$). Due to the rapid deterioration of myocardial function, patients may require IABP or VAD therapy as a bridge to recovery, or a bridge to transplantation. It should be noted that a recurrence of giant cells occurs in 25% of transplanted hearts, but this usually occurs several years after surgery and appears to respond to an increase in immunosuppression.

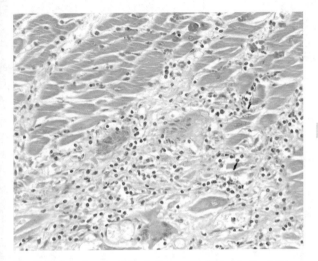

Fig. 19.10 (See colour plate 7) Giant cell myocarditis. The myocardium is being damaged by a marked chronic inflammatory infiltrate that includes prominent multi-nucleated giant cells in the bottom half of the image. Haematoxylin and eosin ×200. Courtesy of Dr Allan McPhaden, Glasgow Royal Infirmary.

Chapter 20

The patient with CHF and preserved LV systolic function

Introduction

The patient presenting with HF in the presence of preserved LV function (PLVEF) presents both a diagnostic and therapeutic challenge. The majority of our evidence-base in HF relates to the management of systolic dysfunction. Controversy exists about the HF with preserved LVEF. Is it diastolic HF and how do we treat it?

The pathophysiology of HF with PLVEF is heterogeneous. It is not merely synonymous with HF due to diastolic dysfunction. Although most patients with HF have abnormalities of both systolic and diastolic function, isolated diastolic function is rare in younger patients. It increases in the elderly. This syndrome is also seen more commonly in women, African-Americans, those with hypertension and in rarer pathologies such as HOCM and restrictive cardiomyopathies (see Table 20.1). The diagnosis is usually more secure when a patient has been hospitalized for heart failure and, for example, there is CXR evidence of pulmonary oedema. This explains, in part, why the mortality rates for hospitalized HF subjects with PLVEF are similar to those of systolic dysfunction, whereas some community cohort studies suggest that this syndrome has a lower mortality rate.

Definition

Can be diagnosed when a patient has:
• Symptoms and/or signs of HF.
• Preserved systolic function at rest.
• Cardiac dysfunction.
• Response to treatment if the diagnosis is in doubt.

Diagnosis

It is important to rule out the other causes of breathlessness that may occur with normal LV systolic function:
• Ischaemia (angina equivalent).
• Respiratory disease.
• Atrial fibrillation (makes systolic dysfunction difficult to measure accurately).
• Valvular disease.
• Anaemia.
• Obesity.
• Deconditioning.
• Pericardial constriction.
• Thyrotoxicosis.

Table 20.1 Clinical characteristics of patients with HF due to systolic or diastolic dysfunction

Characteristic	Systolic HF	Diastolic heart failure
Mean age	61	72
% Female	35	66
% Hypertension	62	85
% CHD	86	45
Exercise time	↓	↓
Peak VO$_2$	↓	↓
Systolic BP	↓ or normal	↑
BNP	↑↑	↑
Morbidity	↑↑	↑↑
Mortality	↑↑	↑

Reproduced from Zile MR, Baicu CF & Bonnema DD. Diastolic heart failure: definitions and terminology. *Prog Cardiovasc Dis* 2005; **47**: 307–13 with permission from Elsevier.

Investigation

Cardiac dysfunction

It is crucial to rule out systolic dysfunction. Part of the confusion surrounding the epidemiology arises from the lack of a definite cut-point for normal systolic function. LVEF is a normally distributed variable.

To attribute this syndrome to 'diastolic heart failure', the following should be present:

- Symptoms and/or signs of HF.
- Presence of normal or only mildly abnormal LV systolic function, that is, LVEF ≥45–50%.
- Evidence of abnormal LV relaxation, diastolic distensibility, or diastolic stiffness.

Invasive investigation

Quantification of impaired relaxation and decreased diastolic compliance, the hallmarks of diastolic dysfunction, is best done invasively (see Fig. 20.1).

Isovolumic relaxation is measured with a high-fidelity micromanometer catheter. This is used to calculate the peak rate of LV pressure decline, peak $(-)$ dP/dt, and the time constant of isovolumic LV pressure decline, τ. When the natural log of LV diastolic pressure is plotted versus time, τ equals the inverse slope of this linear relation. τ is the time that it takes for LV pressure to fall by approximately two-thirds of its initial value. When isovolumic pressure decline is slowed, τ is prolonged and its value increases.

When LV chamber stiffness is increased, the pressure–volume curve shifts to the left, the slope of the dP/dV-versus-pressure relationship becomes steeper, and K_c is increased (the chamber stiffness constant).

As invasive assessment is impractical, hence echocardiography is usually used. However, echo measurements do not directly measure diastolic function and are only markers of impaired diastolic function.

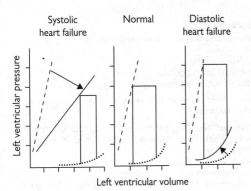

Fig. 20.1 LV pressure–volume loops in systolic heart failure (left), normal (centre), and diastolic HF (right). In SHF, eccentric remodelling leads to increased volumes, the pressure–volume loop being displaced to the right, LVEF is decreased, and the end-systolic pressure–volume line is displaced downward and to the right. In DHF, concentric remodelling results in no significant changes in volumes, LVEF remains normal, chamber stiffness is increased, and the diastolic pressure–volume relation is displaced upwards and to the left. Reproduced from Zile MR, Baicu CF & Bonnema DD. Diastolic heart failure: definitions and terminology. *Prog Cardiovasc Dis* 2005; **47**: 307–13 with permission from Elsevier.

Echocardiography

The most useful echocardiographic measurements are:
- Pulsed wave Doppler.
- Transmitral flow velocities.
- Pulmonary venous flow velocities.
- Mitral annular velocities by tissue Doppler imaging (TDI).

The presence of structural heart disease such as LVH or increased LA size supports the diagnosis.

Three abnormal diastolic filling patterns are recognized by transmitral Doppler (see Fig. 20.2). These patterns represent mild, moderate, and severe DD, respectively:
- Impaired relaxation (E/A < 1).
- Pseudonormalization (intermediate pattern).
- Restrictive (elevated E, short deceleration time, increased E/A ratio)-due to high LAP.

Important points
- The pseudonormal pattern can be distinguished from normal by TDI-decreased E' velocity (E-prime).
- Combining transmitral Doppler with pulmonary venous flow during atrial contraction allows the estimation of LVEDP.
- E/A values are age-dependent and affected by pre- and after-load.

Other investigations

The same investigations should be performed as in HF due to systolic dysfunction.

Although BNP is elevated in patients with HF and PLVEF, the concentration is not as high as in those with systolic dysfunction. BNP concentrations cannot be used to distinguish systolic HF from HF with PLVEF (see Fig. 20.3).

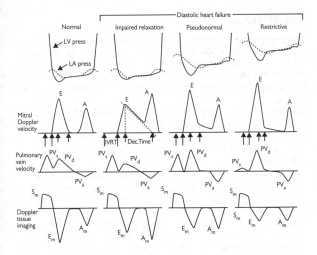

Fig. 20.2 Left ventricular (LV) and left atrial (LA) pressures in diastole, transmitral Doppler LV inflow velocity, pulmonary vein Doppler velocity, and tissue Doppler velocity. A, filling velocity by atrial contraction; A_m, myocardial velocity during filling produced by atrial contraction; Dec. Time, e-wave deceleration time; E, early LV filling velocity; E_m, myocardial velocity during early filling; IVRT, isovolumic relaxation time; PV_a, pulmonary vein velocity resulting from atrial contraction; PV_d, diastolic pulmonary vein velocity; PV_s, systolic pulmonary vein velocity; S_m, myocardial velocity during systole. Reproduced from Zile MR & Brutsaert DL. New concepts in diastolic dysfunction and diastolic heart failure: part I: diagnosis, prognosis, and measurements of diastolic function. *Circulation* 2002; **105**: 1387–93 with permission from Lippincott, Williams and Wilkins.

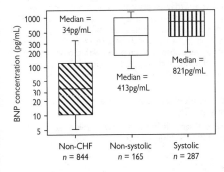

Fig. 20.3 Maisel AS *et al.* Bedside B-type natriuretic peptide in the emergency diagnosis of heart failure with reduced or preserved ejection fraction. Results from the Breathing Not Properly Multinational Study. *J Am Coll Cardiol* 2003; **41**: 2010–7 with permission from Elsevier.

Treatment

The treatment of HF-PLVEF is still largely empirical due to the lack of a secure 'evidence-base'. What trial evidence there is refers to patients with HF and PLVEF-measurements of diastolic function were not usually made. As most HF with PLVEF occurs in the presence of CHD and hypertension, appropriate evidence-based therapies for these should be applied (Table 20.2 and Table 20.3).

Diuretics—should be used for signs of fluid retention. Care should be exercised not to drop pre-load excessively.

Digoxin—the DIG trial enrolled some patients with PLEVF. There was a trend to reduction in the composite endpoint of hospitalization for HF and HF death.

ARBs—the CHARM preserved study randomized 3023 patients with HF and PLVEF to candesartan/placebo. Candesartan was associated with a non-significant trend towards a lower composite endpoint of hospitalization for HF and CV death. There was a reduction in HF hospitalizations.

β-blockers—by a combination of negative inotropy and chrontropy, these should increase diastolic filling time. The SENIORS Trial recruited 752 patients, >70 years of age with HF and randomized them to nebivolol or placebo. One-third of them had a previous hospitalization for HF and PLVEF-LVEF >35%. The reduction in the composite endpoint of death or CV hospitalization seemed to be reduced to a similar extent in those with PLVEF as in those with systolic dysfunction. The target dose of nebivolol was 10mg.

ACEI—should be useful as they increase diastolic distensability and relaxation, in addition, they are antihypertensive agents capable of causing regression of LVH and fibrosis. The PEP-CHF trial randomized 850 HF patients who were at least 70 years of age and had an LVEF of ≥45% and echocardiographic features suggesting possible diastolic dysfunction to receive perindopril at 4mg/day or placebo. Perindopril's effect on the primary endpoint after 1 year fell short of significance overall (p = 0.055). However, there were significant reductions in several subgroups, including patients aged 75 or younger (p = 0.035), or those with a prior MI (p = 0.004). Significant improvements were observed compared with the placebo group in some secondary endpoints, including the proportion of patients in NYHA functional class 1 (p < 0.03) and change in 6-minute-walk distance (p = 0.02).

Verapamil—has been suggested due to its negative inotropic and chronotropic effects, especially in HCM.

Future—there are several large RCTs underway in this area; TOPCAT (Spironolactone) and I-PRESERVE (Irbesartan).

Table 20.2 Randomized controlled trials enrolling patients with HF and PLVEF

Study	Drug	Target dose (mg)	n	LVEF (%)	Mean follow-up (months)
DIG study	Digoxin	0.25*	988	>45	37
CHARM	Candesartan	32	850	≥45	26
PEP-CHF	Perindopril	4	3023	>40	36.6

*Digoxin dose was titrated by an algorithm (range 0.125–0.5mg), median dose at randomization was 0.25mg.

Reproduced from: The effect of digoxin on mortality and morbidity in patients with heart failure. The Digitalis Investigation Group. *N Engl J Med* 1997; **336**: 525–33 with permission from Massacheussets Medical Society.

Table 20.3 Results of treatment in RCTs in patients with HF and PLVEF

Study	HR (95% CI) for 1° end point, p value	HF hospitalization
DIG study	0.82 (0.63–1.07, p = 0.136	0.79 (0.59–1.04), p = 0.094
PEP CHF	0.92 (0.70–1.21), p = 0.545	0.63 (0.41–0.97), p = 0.033
CHARM	0.86 (0.74–1.00), p = 0.051	0.84 (0.7–1.00), p = 0.047

Reproduced from: The effect of digoxin on mortality and morbidity in patients with heart failure. The Digitalis Investigation Group. *N Engl J Med* 1997; **336**: 525–33 with permission from Massacheussets Medical Society.

Primary endpoints

Dig Ancillary Study: HF mortality or HF hospitalization

PEP-CHF: All cause mortality or unplanned HF hospitalization

CHARM; CV mortality or HF hospitalization

Key references

Ahmed A *et al.* Effects of digoxin on morbidity and mortality in diastolic heart failure: the ancillary digitalis investigation group trial. *Circulation* 2006; **114**: 397–403.

Cleland JG *et al.* The perindopril in elderly people with chronic heart failure (PEP-CHF) study. *Eur Heart J* 2006; **27**: 2338–45.

Yusuf S *et al.* Effects of candesartan in patients with chronic heart failure and preserved left-ventricular ejection fraction: the CHARM-Preserved Trial. *Lancet* 2003; **362**: 778–81.

Chapter 21

The patient with CHF and sleep-disordered breathing

Introduction

There are two types of sleep-disordered breathing (SDB) (see Fig. 21.1):
- Obstructive sleep apnoea (OSA).
- Central sleep apnoea (CSA).

Both can coexist in HF patients.

Characteristics

Obstructive sleep apnoea–hypopnoea

OSA is caused by collapse of the pharyngeal airway during sleep. This leads to
- Absent air flow.
- Paradoxical chest wall and abdominal movement.
- Arterial oxygen desaturation.

OSA is an independent risk factor for developing hypertension. OSA patients have a higher prevalence of CHD and may accelerate progression of coexisting CHF.

Risk factors for OSA are:
- Male sex.
- Obesity (♂).
- Age >60 years for women.

Central sleep-apnoea–hypopnoea

CSA is caused by reduced efferent activity to the respiratory muscles. It is terminated by arousal from sleep. It is probably a consequence of HF. During CSA there is:
- Absence of chest wall movement.
- Arterial desaturation.

There are several variant forms of CSA, including Cheyne–Stokes respiration. This describes crescendo–decrescendo oscillation of tidal volume, with episodes of hyperventilation and apnoea/hypopnoea.

Risk factors for CSA are:
- Male sex.
- Age >60 years.
- AF.
- An awake pCO_2 of ≤38mmHg (5.1kPa).

Prevalence

Early studies suggested that SDB occurs in up to 50% of patients with moderate to severe HF. The predominant type is CSA. More recent work in a cohort of patients with mild HF on modern HF treatment showed a prevalence of 53%, two-thirds had CSA (Fig. 21.2).

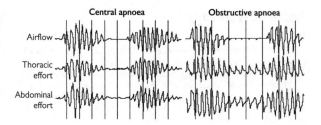

Fig. 21.1 Typical central and obstructive apnoea events obtained from a patient with CHF. During the central apnoea, there is absence of air flow and absence of both chest wall (thoracic effort) and abdominal movement (abdominal effort). During the obstructive event, there is absence of air flow together with continued, but paradoxical, chest wall and abdominal movement. Reproduced from Vazir A *et al. Br J Cardiol* 2005; **12**: 219–23. with permission from The British Journal of Cardiology.

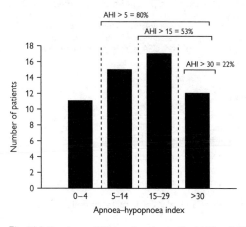

Fig. 21.2 Prevalence of SDB in male patients with mild HF and LVSD. Vazir A *et al. Eur J Heart Fail* 2007; **9**: 243–50 with permission from Elsevier.

Pathophysiology

OSA

Increased inspiratory efforts against an occluded pharynx during apnoeas generate enhanced negative intrathoracic pressure that increases LV transmural pressure, and, therefore, after-load. It also increases venous return, distending the RV, and displaces the IV septum in diastole - impairing LV filling. The intermittent hypoxia may impair cardiac contractility and precipitate ischaemia. The arousal from sleep, hypoxia and hypercapnoea trigger SNS outflow with its resultant deleterious effects in HF. This enhanced SNS activity and decreased parasympathetic modulation of HR result in hypertension during the daytime.

CSA

CSA is thought to be related to chronic hypocapnoea due to increased LVEDP and pulmonary congestion that may provoke hyperventilation in HF. This hyperventilation reduces pCO_2 below the apnoeic threshold. When this happens chronically, there is enhanced chemosensitivity, so the resultant fall in pO_2 and rise in pCO_2 with apnoea causes ventilatory overshoot leading to a further reduction in pCO_2 and hence cyclical alternation of apnoea and hyperventilation. There are intermittent SNS and blood pressure surges. This enhanced SNS activity may decrease survival in patients with HF and CSA and lead to progression of the syndrome.

Symptoms

In the general population, OSA is associated with, obesity, snoring, and daytime fatigue, somnolence and daytime headaches. Most HF patients do not display typical symptoms of SDB, hence diagnosis on clinical grounds is difficult.

Diagnosis
- 10–15 apnoea–hypopnoea episodes per hour of sleep (apnoea–hypopnoea index (AHI)).
- Division into OSA or CSA if >50% of episodes are in either category.

Investigation
- The gold standard is nocturnal polysomnography. It involves an EEG, ECG, EMG, and electro-oculography. Nasal air flow/pressure and abdominal and chest wall movements are measured, as well as pulse oximetry. It is expensive, time-consuming and not widely available.
- Respiratory screening devices that measure oro-nasal air flow, chest and abdominal wall movement and pulse oximetry usually suffice,-they have a high sensitivity and specificity for detecting SDB in HF patients.
- Home pulse oximetry can also be used with a sensitivity of 85% and specificity of 93% for detecting SDB in HF.

Key references

Arzt M & Bradley TD. Treatment of sleep apnea in heart failure. *Am J Respir Crit Care Med* 2006; **173**: 1300–8.

Vazir A et al. Sleep-disordered breathing and heart failure: an oppurtunity missed? *Br J Cardiol* 2005; **12**: 219–23.

Vazir A et al. A high prevalence of sleep-disordered breathing in men with mild symptomatic chronic heart failure due to left ventricular systolic dysfunction. *Eur J Heart Fail* 2007; **9**: 243–50.

Treatment

OSA

Treatment with CPAP via a nasal or facemask is well established. It reduces episodes of apnoea–hypopnoea, the number of arousals and daytime somnolence.

In HF, a small RCT has shown that CPAP used for 1 month:
• Improved LVEF by 9%.
• Decreased daytime HR and BP.

Another study in 55 CHF patients showed that 3 months of CPAP increased LVEF by 5% and reduced sympathetic activity and improved quality of life.

CSA

The treatment of CSA remains unclear.

Drugs

Studies have shown that
• Optimization of CHF therapy may improve apnoea–hypopnoea index (AHI).
• Theophylline reduces AHI, but is not recommended due to its deleterious cardiac effects.
• Acetazolamide also reduces AHI significantly. Its long-term effects on cardiac function are unknown.
• Benzodiazepines have shown mixed results.
• Opiates may reduce AHI by their effects on chemosensitivity.
• Continuous nasal oxygen during sleep for 1 week reduced AHI and improved HF symptoms in one study; another study showed no effects.
• CO_2 therapy has been tried; it reduces AHI but may increase arousal and is poorly tolerated.

CPAP

Small studies have shown:
• Improvements in cardiac function.
• Reduced sympathetic activity.
• Improved QOL.

The recent CANPAP study randomized 300 patients with CSA to CPAP versus placebo. It was terminated early. CPAP:
• Did not reduce mortality.
• Improved 6-minute walk time.
• Increased LVEF by 2.2%.

At this time CPAP cannot be advised for the treatment of CSA in CHF.

Respiratory support devices

Small studies with bi-level non-invasive ventilation and adaptive servo-ventilation (ASV) have shown improvements in central apnoeas. They await more definitive testing.

Pacing

An early study using atrial overdrive pacing reduced AHI by 50%. However, this was not replicated in later studies. More recently, two studies using CRT have shown improvements in AHI, NYHA class, exercise tolerance, and LVEF.

Key references

Bradley TD et al. Continuous positive airway pressure for central sleep apnea and heart failure. N Engl J Med 2005; **353**: 2025–33.

Mansfield DR et al. Controlled trial of continuous positive airway pressure in obstructive sleep apnea and heart failure. Am J Respir Crit Care Med 2004; **169**; 361–6.

Chapter 22

The patient with CHF and cancer

Introduction

Cancer can occur at any age. It can be associated with heart failure in three ways:
• HF as a consequence of cancer.
• HF as a result of the treatment of cancer.
• Established HF requiring treatment of malignancy.

The treatment of many cancers involves the use of potent chemotherapeutic agents and/or radiotherapy. These treatment modalities have radically improved survival in many cancers. However, the cost in the long term may include cardiotoxicity resulting in arrhythmias, coronary artery stenosis, or myocardial fibrosis, or necrosis with resultant heart failure.

It has been increasingly recognized that the toxic cardiac effects are more often seen in multi-agent regimes. There is a synergistic cardiotoxicity associated with combining chemotherapy and mediastinal radiotherapy. The cardiac side effects of the therapy may take years to manifest. This raises difficult questions in considering whether there may be a role for the use of heart failure medications as prophylaxis, and in how best to monitor for cardiotoxicity.

Malignancies that are more commonly associated with CHF
• Breast cancer.
• Lymphoma, especially Hodgkin's lymphoma.
• Lung.
• Leukaemia requiring haemopoietic cell transplant.
• Testicular germ cell tumours.

Heart failure as a consequence of malignancy
The majority of malignancies affecting the heart are secondary to a remote primary disease. In a study of 1900 patients dying of cancer, 8% had cardiac metastases. The development of cardiomegaly, a new murmur, or dysrhythmia may be the first sign of cardiac metastases. Heart failure may be due to cardiac or pericardial infiltration. Direct invasion or cardiac infiltration can result from primary mediastinal tumours and lung cancer.

Primary cardiac tumours include both benign and malignant lesions. Over 75% are benign. Myxomas, lipomas, and fibromas may cause symptoms of heart failure as a consequence of valvular obstruction. Malignant sarcomas have a poor prognosis, and may be associated with heart failure due to myocardial infiltration.

Malignant pericardial effusions may cause symptoms of heart failure by restricting cardiac filling. They can present with haemodynamic compromise as cardiac tamponade. In the acute setting, the symptoms can be relieved with pericardiocentesis and placement of a pericardial drain. The drain is usually left in place until the effusion is drained completely. This is confirmed with echocardiography and that <30mL has drained in the 24 hours prior to removal. This may require the drain to be in place for 2–3 days.

The role of pericardial sclerosis by the instillation of a sclerosing agent is debatable. Initial studies used tetracycline, but further small studies have used a wide range of chemotherapeutic agents including bleomycin. There does not appear to be evidence of benefit from pericardial sclerosis over simple pericardial drainage. Patients may have significant side effects from the instillation of the sclerosing agent, including chest pain and atrial arrhythmias.

Recurrent pericardial effusions may be managed by the creation of a pericardial window. Studies suggest that the sub-xiphoid approach for pericardiotomy was well tolerated with minimal complications. This approach avoids the need for thoracotomy and lengthy procedure time, which may be inappropriate given the prognosis of the primary disease.

Cardiac effects of cancer therapies

Radiotherapy

Studies of the effect of mediastinal radiation in animal models have demonstrated that there are three distinct phases to the myocardial reaction:
- Acute phase—neutrophil infiltration of all myocardial layers.
- Latent phase—no additional damage seen.
- Late phase—fibrotic reaction of the pericardium and myocardium; endovascular damage with resultant capillary obstruction.

The clinical manifestations of radiotherapy include:
- Pericarditis.
  - Acute.
  - Chronic.
  - Pericardial constriction.
- Pancarditis including valve dysfunction.
- Coronary artery stenosis.
  - Most commonly ostial stenosis of left anterior descending artery.
- Dysrhythmias.
- Cardiomyopathy.

Strategies to reduce the cardiotoxic impact of radiotherapy include:
- Modification of cardiac risk factors.
  - Smoking.
  - Lipid profile.
- Tangential radiation beams.
- Respiratory gating.
- Limitation of radiation fraction size.

Management of radiation pericarditis

Clinical evidence of pericarditis may develop acutely after therapy, but more commonly presents more than a year later. Approximately, 50% of patients will develop severe constrictive pericarditis requiring surgical pericardiectomy. The operative mortality is significant between 6 and 21%, and the 5-year post-operative survival is poor between 1 and 27%.

Chemotherapy

The majority of patients receiving standard doses of chemotherapy do not suffer any adverse cardiac effect. However, these patients are at risk of developing cardiotoxicity. The incidence and severity of cardiotoxicity depend on:
- Patient's age.
- Presence of coexisting cardiac diseases.
- Type of drugs used.
- Dose and schedule employed.
- Radiotherapy—particularly mediastinal.

When considering the cardiotoxic effects of chemotherapeutic agents, it is worthwhile considering two classes of agents: anthracycline-like agents and non-anthracycline agents.

Chemotherapy agents with known cardiotoxicity
- Anthracyclines including doxorubicin.
- Trastuzumab (Herceptin®) and alemtuzumab.
- Taxanes including paclitaxel and docetaxel.
- *Vinca* alkaloids including vincristine.
- 5-fluorouracil and capecitabine.
- Fludarabine in combination with melphalan.
- Cyclophosphamide and ifosfamide.
- Cisplatin.
- Mitomycin-C.
- Interferon-α.

Key reference

Bertog SC *et al.* Constrictive pericarditis: etiology and cause-specific survival after pericardiectomy. *J Am Coll Cardiol* 2004; **43**: 1445–52.

Anthracycline-like agents

This group includes doxorubicin, daunorubicin, epirubicin, and also the anthraquinone mitoxantrone. These agents are highly effective in the management of a wide range of malignancies. Unfortunately, they are also among the most frequent causes of chemotherapy-related cardiotoxicity that may result in severe, irreversible, and sometimes fatal cardiomyopathy.

Anthracyclines work by inserting into the DNA of replicating cells causing DNA fragmentation and disrupting the action of polymerases. As cardiomyocytes do not actively replicate, it is postulated that the cardiotoxic effect is related to the production of free radicals and increased oxidative stress with resultant cardiomyocyte damage and fibrotic replacement. In addition to the dilated cardiomyopathy that may result from myocardial necrosis, anthracyclines are associated with a risk of dysrhythmias and coronary artery disease.

There are three phases of anthracycline cardiotoxicity:
- Acute toxicity.
  - Rare and usually not associated with clinical signs.
  - ECG changes including increased QTc, ventricular and supraventricular ectopics.
  - LV systolic dysfunction and rises in BNP.
- Early toxicity.
  - Peak time for presentation with heart failure is 3 months post-dose.
- Late toxicity.
  - Heart failure may occur more than 10 years after chemotherapy.

Risk factors have been identified in the development of cardiotoxicity:
- Cumulative dose.
  - Doxorubicin   >500mg/m^2
  - Daunorubicin   >500mg/m^2
  - Epirubicin   >900mg/m^2
- Patient age.
  - Age >65 years—possibly due to underlying ischaemic heart disease.
  - Children.
- Radiotherapy.
- Concomitant chemotherapy.
  - For example, cyclophosphamide, trastuzumab, and taxanes.

Risk reduction strategies include:
- Surveillance.
  - Echocardiography at baseline and if requiring additional doses.
- Continuous infusion rather than bolus.
- Liposomal formulations.
- Dexrazoxane—an EDTA-like chelating agent (see opposite).
- Biomarkers.
  - Serum Tn-T and -I may be an early indicator for at-risk patients.
  - NT-BNP may be useful to screen for asymptomatic ventricular dysfunction.

Suggested doxorubicin cardiac monitoring algorithm

Schwartz RG et al. Congestive heart failure and left ventricular dysfunction complicating doxorubicin therapy. Seven-year experience using serial radionuclide angiocardiography. *Am J Med* 1987; **82**: 1109–18.

If baseline LVEF >50%

Stop doxorubicin therapy if LVEF reduced by ≥10% + LVEF ≤50%.

- Repeat LVEF after 250–300mg/m^2.
- Repeat LVEF after 400mg/m^2 if:
  - Heart disease
  - Radiation exposure
  - Cyclophosphamide therapy.
- Otherwise repeat after 450mg/m^2.

If baseline LVEF <50%

Stop doxorubicin if LVEF reduced by ≥10% +/or LVEF ≤30%.

- Do not initiate therapy if LVEF ≤30%.
- Assess LVEF before each dose.

Dexrazoxane

A meta-analysis has demonstrated that dexrazoxane reduces the incidence of heart failure in patients receiving anthracyclines if started either at the initiation of therapy or after a cumulative dose of 300mg/m^2. There are suggestions that dexrazoxane may reduce the efficacy of chemotherapy or enhance the anthracycline-associated myelosuppression.

Guidelines for the use of dexrazoxane suggest that it be considered in patients with metastatic disease with a cumulative dose of >300mg/m^2 of doxorubicin, who require further doses. It may also be considered for use in patients receiving epirubicin.

Key references

Schuchter LM et al. 2002 update of recommendations for the use of chemotherapy and radio-therapy protectants: clinical practice guidelines of the American Society of Clinical Oncology. *J Clin Oncol* 2002; **20**: 2895–903.

van Dalen EC et al. Cardioprotective interventions for patients receiving anthracyclines. *Cochrane Database Syst Rev* 2005; **25**: CD003917.

Non-anthracycline agents

Heart failure may result from direct cardiotoxicity, secondary to chemo-therapy-related myocardial infarction, or due to pericardial effusion.

Direct cardiotoxicity is associated with:
- Alkylating agents.
  - Cisplatin.
  - Ifosfamide.
  - Mitomycin.
- Antimetabolites.
  - Cytarabine.
  - Pentostatin.
- Antimicrotubules.
  - Taxanes including paclitaxel (especially if combined with anthracycline).
- Biological agents.
  - Monoclonal antibodies including bevacizumab and trastuzumab.
  - Interferon-α.
- Amsacrine—topoisomerase II inhibitor.
- Imatinib (Glivec®)—specific tyrosine kinase inhibitor.
- Tretinoin.

Myocardial infarction may be due to coronary artery spasm:
- Alkylating agents.
  - Cisplatin.
- Antimetabolites.
  - Capecitabine.
  - Fluorouracil.
- Antimicrotubules.
  - *Vinca* alkaloids.
- Biological agents.
  - Interferon-α.

Pericardial effusion may be related to therapy with:
- Alkylating agents.
  - Busulfan—which may also cause endomyocardial fibrosis.
- Cyclophosphamide.
- Imatinib.
- Tretinoin.

Key references

Kerkela R et al. Cardiotoxicity of the cancer therapeutic agent imatinib mesylate. *Nat Med* 2006; **12**: 908–16.
Yeh ET et al. Cardiovascular complications of cancer therapy: diagnosis, pathogenesis, and management. *Circulation* 2004; **109**: 3122–31.

Trastuzumab (Herceptin®) and CHF

Recent developments in the management of breast cancer have offered improved survival particularly for early-stage breast cancer. Patients are assessed for the need for adjuvant systemic therapy in addition to surgery. The determinants of the need for, and nature of, adjuvant therapy include:

• Estimated risk of disease recurrence.
• Pathology of the presenting breast tumour (hormone-responsive state).
• Overexpression of HER-2/neu cell surface molecule.

The possible options for adjuvant therapy include hormone therapy, chemotherapy that may include anthracyclines, cyclophosphamide, and taxanes, and the anti-HER2 monoclonal antibody trastuzumab.

Trastuzumab is also effective in the management of metastatic breast cancer that overexpresses HER-2/neu. Therefore, there is a sizeable population of women who may benefit from this therapy. However, trastuzumab has significant potential cardiotoxicity including both symptomatic and asymptomatic left ventricular systolic dysfunction and arrhythmias that does not appear to be dose-related. Unlike the anthracyclines, this may not be reversible heart failure. The likelihood of developing heart failure is increased if trastuzumab is combined with anthracyclines and/or taxanes or cyclophosphamide. Other risk factors for the development of cardio-myopathy include previous anthracyclines use, age >50 years, previous cardiac disease, and hyperlipidaemia.

The mechanism of the trastuzumab-induced heart failure is not entirely clear; however, there is evidence that Neuregulin-1 beta, a ligand of the HER-2/neu receptor, may attenuate doxorubicin-induced alterations of excitation-contraction coupling. Further evidence suggests that the activation of this receptor improves systolic function in a number of cardio-myopathies. This may explain the increased incidence of heart failure in those receiving multi-modality therapy.

The experience with trastuzumab to date has suggested guidelines for its use. Careful initial cardiac assessment is required including documentation of LVEF (either by radionuclide ventriculography or echo). Therapy should not be commenced if the LVEF is <55%. At each subsequent visit, the patient is re-examined and formal re-assessment of LVEF is warranted if:

• Rise in heart rate from baseline.
  ◦ Baseline HR <80bpm and increases to >90bpm.
  ◦ Baseline HR >80 but <100bpm and increases to >100bpm.
  ◦ Baseline HR >100bpm and increases to >120bpm.
• Body weight increased by >2kg in 1 week.
• Spontaneous report of exertional breathlessness.

Routine repeat assessment of LVEF should occur every 3 months during therapy.

Trastuzumab should not be given if baseline assessment identifies:
- LVEF <55%.
- Uncontrolled hypertension.
- High-risk uncontrolled arrhythmias.
- Angina requiring medication.
- Clinically significant valve disease.
- Clinical history of heart failure.
- Evidence of transmural MI on ECG.

If LVEF falls by >10% and to below 50%:
- Suspend therapy with trastuzumab.
- Commence heart failure therapy including ACE inhibitors + β-blockers.
- Re-assess LVEF.
  - If improved, consider re-starting trastuzumab.
  - If static or worse, no further trastuzumab.

Key references

Keefe DL. Trastuzumab-associated cardiotoxicity. *Cancer* 2002; 95: 1592–600.

Liu X et al. Neuregulin-1/erbB-activation improves cardiac function and survival in models of ischemic, dilated, and viral cardiomyopathy. *J Am Coll Cardiol* 2006; **48**: 1438–47.

NICE technology appraisal guidance number 107. Published August 2006.

Schuchter LM, Hensley ML, Meropol NJ et al. Neuregulin-1 beta attenuates doxorubicin-induced alterations of excitation-contraction coupling and reduces oxidative stress in adult rat cardiomyocytes. *J Mol Cell Cardiol* 2006; September e-pub ahead of print.

Suter TM, Cook-Bruns N & Barton C. Cardiotoxicity associated with trastuzumab (Herceptin) therapy in the treatment of metastatic breast cancer. *Breast* 2004; **13**: 173–83.

Measures to minimize the cardiotoxic effects

Patients who may need to receive chemotherapeutic agents that are associated with potential cardiotoxicity should be screened prior to initiation of therapy. Screening should include:

- History.
  - Cardiovascular risk factors including smoking and hyperlipidaemia.
  - Angina or previous myocardial infarction.
  - Previous clinical heart failure.
- Examination.
  - Hypertension.
  - Heart failure.
- Previous chemotherapy and radiotherapy.
- Planned concomitant chemotherapy and radiotherapy.

Risk factors should be addressed, and the management of hypertension and heart failure initiated.

Baseline assessment for those with a positive finding during screening should include documentation of LVEF. A clinical decision should then be made balancing the risk of therapy-related cardiotoxicity with the potential benefit. There may be specific measures that can be taken to reduce cardiotoxicity, for example, Dexrazoxane, liposomal formulations or infusion or bolus regimes. Clinical need for the use of therapy with potential cardiotoxicity should prompt the cardiologist to strive to pre-optimize the patient and then a careful screening programme should be tailored to the individual patient.

Screening for the development of cardiotoxicity should be performed at the clinic follow-up. Symptoms or signs suggestive of developing heart failure should prompt re-assessment of the LVEF. If there is evidence of a decline in LVEF, then the planned therapy may need to be modified and referral made to a cardiologist for management of heart failure. There may be a role for cardiac biomarkers in screening for LV dysfunction. There is preliminary evidence of a role for both Troponin (T or I) and NT-pro-BNP.

The role of 'prophylactic' heart failure medications for particularly potent combined regimes of chemotherapy and/or radiotherapy is not clear. In asymptomatic anthracycline-related left ventricular dysfunction, there are small trials assessing the effect of ACE inhibitors in the survivors of childhood cancers. Whilst they do appear to be beneficial, they do not prevent progressive disease. There is evidence of benefit of traditional heart failure medications in symptomatic heart failure related to cancer therapy. There may be a role for cardiac transplantation in the management of cancer therapy-related CHF if the presentation is remote to the diagnosis of malignancy and the therapy has been curative.

Key reference

Ng R, Better N & Green MD. Anticancer agents and cardiotoxicity. *Semin Oncol* 2006; **33**: 2–14.

Section III

Acute heart failure

Acute heart failure: from definition to diagnosis

Definition

Acute heart failure (AHF) is the rapid onset of symptoms attributable to abnormal cardiac function. It may occur *de novo* or as an acute decompensation of CHF. The European Society of Cardiology (ESC) has classified acute heart failure according to its clinical presentation.

- Acute decompensated heart failure, which does not fulfil the criteria for cardiogenic shock, pulmonary oedema or hypertensive crisis.
- Hypertensive AHF, with signs and symptoms of heart failure accompanied by high blood pressure but with relatively preserved left ventricular function.
- Pulmonary oedema, accompanied by severe respiratory distress, crepitations and orthopnoea, with O_2 saturation usually <90% on room air.
- Cardiogenic shock is defined as an evidence of tissue hypoperfusion induced by heart failure after the correction of pre-load. Cardiogenic shock is usually characterized by reduced blood pressure (systolic BP <90mmHg or a drop of mean arterial pressure >30mmHg) and/or low urine output (<0.5mL/kg/hour), with a pulse rate >60/minute with or without evidence of organ congestion.
- High output failure is characterized by high cardiac output, usually with high heart rate with warm peripheries, pulmonary congestion, and sometimes with low BP as in septic shock. Causes include
  - Hyperthyroidism.
  - Anaemia.
  - Beri-beri.
  - Paget's disease.
  - Psoriasis.
- Right heart failure is characterized by low output syndrome with increased jugular venous pressure, increased liver size, and hypotension. Causes include
  - Right ventricular myocardial infarction.
  - Chronic lung disease.
  - Significant pulmonary embolism.
  - Cardiac tamponade.
  - Valve disease.
  - Congenital heart disease.
  - Arrhythmogenic right ventricular cardiomyopathy.

Key reference

Nieminen MS *et al.* Executive summary of the guidelines on the diagnosis and treatment of acute heart failure: the Task Force on Acute Heart Failure of the European Society of Cardiology. *Eur Heart J* 2005; **26**: 384–416.

Epidemiology

The median age of an acute heart failure presentation is 75 years in a US Registry. The aetiology will vary with geography; however, ischaemic heart disease accounts for 60–70% of patients, particularly in the elderly population. In younger subjects, AHF frequently results from the many forms of dilated cardiomyopathy, arrhythmia, congenital or valvular heart disease, or myocarditis.

The ageing population, combined with the improved survival after acute myocardial infarction, has led to a marked increase in the number of patients currently living with chronic heart failure. Consequently, there has been an increase in hospitalizations for decompensated heart failure. The mortality and morbidity of AHF is high, with a risk of 30-day mortality of up to 30%. Furthermore, the 30-day risk of readmission is as high as 60%. The prognosis of AHF is particularly poor following acute myocardial infarction.

According to the ESC, the management of heart failure consumes 1–2% of health care expenditure in European countries, with around 75% relating to inpatient care.

Aetiology

There are many causes for acute heart failure. They include:
- Decompensation of pre-existing chronic heart failure.
- Acute coronary syndrome.
- Bradyarrhythmias or tachyarrhythmias.
- Non-cardiovascular precipitating factors (e.g. sepsis).
- Poor compliance with medical treatment or fluid restriction (15–64%).
- High output syndromes (e.g. sepsis, thyrotoxicosis).
- Acute valvular regurgitation (e.g. rupture of chordae tendinae).
- Hypertensive crisis.
- Myocarditis.
- Cardiac tamponade.
- Aortic dissection.
- Post-partum cardiomyopathy.

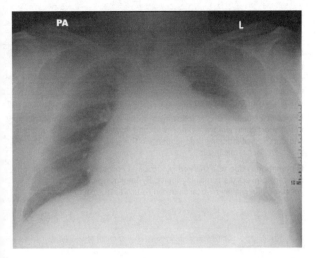

Fig. 23.1 CXR of a pericardial effusion.

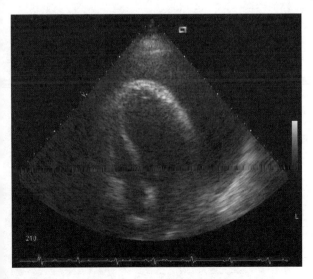

Fig. 23.2 An echocardiogram of a large pericardial effusion with significant collapse of the right ventricle.

Pathophysiology of AHF

The key feature of AHF is a failure of the heart to maintain circulation required for peripheral perfusion.

Many causes of AHF are partly, or wholly, reversible. As ischaemia is the most common precipitant of AHF, it is important to appreciate that cardiac dysfunction due to stunning or hibernation can return to normal when appropriately treated.

Myocardial stunning occurs following prolonged ischaemia, and may persist in the short term even when normal blood flow is restored. The intensity and duration of stunning is dependent on the severity and duration of the preceding ischaemic insult.

Hibernation is due to a marked reduction in coronary blood flow despite the cardiomyocytes remaining intact. By improving blood flow and oxygenation, hibernating myocardium can return to normal function.

Clinical features of AHF

AHF is a clinical syndrome, as a consequence of increased pre-load, increased after-load, or a reduced cardiac output. This results in tissue hypoperfusion and congestion.

Symptoms
- Breathlessness.
- Orthopnoea/PND.
- Oedema.
- Fatigue.

Signs
- Tachycardia (or bradycardia; if this is the cause or, patient β-blocked).
- Thready rapid pulse.
- Hypotensive (or hypertensive in cases of hypertensive crisis).
- Elevated JVP.
- S_3 gallop.
- Murmurs.
- Oliguria.
- Hepatomegaly.
- Ascites.
- Peripheral/sacral oedema.
- Pulmonary congestion with crepitations.
- Increased body mass.

Haemodynamics
Fig. 23.3 describes four haemodynamic categories that the patient may present in: warm and dry, warm and wet, cold and dry, and cold and wet. Patients presenting wet and warm or wet and cold are at the highest risk of death or need of urgent cardiac transplantation.

Killip classification
The Killip classification was designed to provide a clinical estimate of the severity of myocardial derangement in the treatment of acute myocardial infarction.

Stage I   No heart failure. No clinical signs of cardiac decompensation
Stage II   Heart failure. Diagnostic criteria include crepitations and S_3 gallop
Stage III Severe heart failure. Frank pulmonary oedema with crepitations throughout the lung fields
Stage IV   Cardiogenic shock. Signs include hypotension (SBP <90mmHg) and evidence of peripheral vasoconstriction such as oliguria and cyanosis

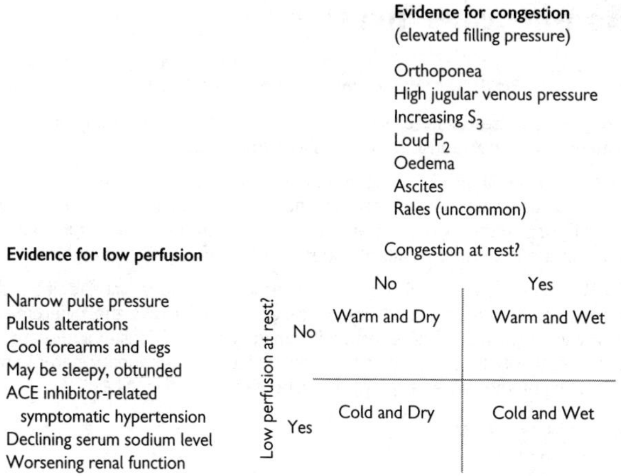

Evidence for congestion
(elevated filling pressure)

Orthoponea
High jugular venous pressure
Increasing S_3
Loud P_2
Oedema
Ascites
Rales (uncommon)

Evidence for low perfusion

Congestion at rest?

		No	Yes
	No	Warm and Dry	Warm and Wet
	Yes	Cold and Dry	Cold and Wet

Narrow pulse pressure
Pulsus alterations
Cool forearms and legs
May be sleepy, obtunded
ACE inhibitor-related
  symptomatic hypertension
Declining serum sodium level
Worsening renal function

Low perfusion at rest?

Fig. 23.3 2-minute assessment of haemodynamic profile. Reproduced from Nohria *et al.* Medical management of advanced heart failure. *JAMA* 2002; **287**: 628–40 (on page 630) with permission from the American Medical Association.

Key references

Nohria A *et al.* Clinical assessment identifies hemodynamic profiles that predict outcomes in patients admitted with heart failure. *J Am Coll Cardiol* 2003; **41**: 1797–804.

Non-invasive investigation

The diagnosis of AHF is based on the symptoms and signs mentioned earlier, supported by the following investigations (Fig. 23.4).

SaO₂—the pulse oximeter should be used continuously on any unstable patient. It may not transduce in the shocked patient.

ECG—a normal ECG is uncommon in acute heart failure. The ECG should be used to assess the rhythm, and may help determine the aetiology of AHF (e.g. acute myocardial infarction). Continuous ECG monitoring is appropriate in these critically ill patients to identify cardiac arrhythmia.

CXR—to evaluate pre-existing chest or cardiac conditions (cardiac size and shape) and to assess pulmonary congestion. CXR allows the differential diagnosis of left heart failure from inflammatory or infectious lung diseases. A CT scan of the chest may be used to identify pulmonary pathology (including pulmonary embolism) or aortic dissection (Fig. 23.4).

Laboratory tests

Recommended
- Urea and electrolytes.
- Liver function tests.
- Albumin.
- Thyroid function.
- Full blood count.
- Arterial blood gas analysis.
- Plasma BNP/NT-pro-BNP.
- INR (if patient anticoagulated or in severe heart failure).
- CRP.
- Blood glucose.
- TnI/TnT.

Consider
- Measurement of mixed venous O_2 saturation from a central vein estimates the total body oxygen supply–demand balance. A SvO_2 <70% is indicative of a low output state and inadequate tissue perfusion.
- D-dimers (may be falsely elevated).
- Urine analysis.

Echocardiography—an essential tool to evaluate regional and global ventricular function, as well as an assessment of valvular dysfunction. Echo is also used to diagnose pericardial pathology, post-myocardial infarction VSDs.

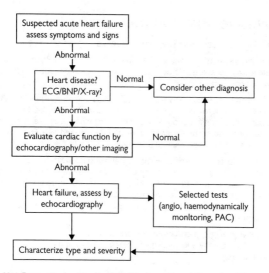

Fig. 23.4 Diagnostic algorithm for AHF. Nieminen MS *et al.* Reproduced from Executive summary of the guidelines on the diagnosis and treatment of acute heart failure: the Task Force on Acute Heart Failure of the European Society of Cardiology. *Eur Heart J* 2005; **26**: 384–416 with permission from Oxford University Press.

Invasive investigation

Urinary catheter with hourly volumes

Central venous pressure (CVP)—(📖 Chapter 25) Right ventricular preload can be assessed from the CVP, with caution needed in the context of significant tricuspid regurgitation.

Pulmonary artery catheter (PAC)—(📖 Chapter 26) In critically ill patients, or where the diagnosis is in doubt, a PAC can be helpful. As well as giving an estimation of left ventricular filling pressure, it can also be used to document cardiac output, pulmonary and systemic vascular resistance, and the presence of an intra-cardiac shunt.

Invasive arterial monitoring—to allow beat–beat blood pressure monitoring and titration of inotropic/vasodilator therapy. In addition, this facilitates close monitoring of acid–base status. An intra-aortic balloon pump (📖 Chapter 28) incorporates these features. In the era of radial approach coronary angiography, it is best to avoid the right radial artery, where possible.

Coronary angiography—in the presence of an acute coronary syndrome, angiography and subsequent revascularization has been shown to reduce mortality.

Chapter 24

Acute heart failure: management

Introduction

Having established the diagnosis of acute heart failure, the immediate aim is to implement resuscitation. If there is any evidence of airway compromise, including exhaustion or reduced conscious level, an anaesthetic opinion should be sought as a matter of urgency. Thereafter measures should be instituted to stabilize and optimize breathing and circulation, aiming for a systolic pressure >90mmHg to ensure adequate coronary perfusion.

Much of the therapy for AHF has not been subjected to rigorous clinical trials, but due to the established nature of these drugs it would be difficult to ethically design a trial that might replace them with placebo. Therefore, clinical guidelines incorporate and advocate their use. There are, however, newer therapies and technologies that are currently under investigation.

It should be recognized that the patient with AHF is critically ill and therefore should be cared for by expert staff in a high-dependency environment. Particular care should be taken to minimize the risk of infection and to ensure adequate nutrition with normoglycaemia in diabetic patients.

An algorithm summarizing the treatment for AHF is shown in Fig. 24.1. The various aspects will be discussed in more detail both in this chapter and in the detailed pharmacology (📖 Section V).

It is also important to avoid certain drugs, which have been shown to worsen outcome in AHF:
- Calcium antagonists (with the exception of amlodipine and felodipine).
- NSAIDS.
- Steroids.
- Metformin.
- Tricyclic antidepressants.

The other common issue in the management of AHF is the role of β-adrenoreceptor antagonists. Patients established on this therapy who are admitted due to worsening heart failure should be maintained on their current dose, unless inotropic support is needed. The dose could be reduced if signs of excessive dosage are suspected (that is, bradycardia and hypotension). However, there is no role for the initiation of β-adrenoreceptor antagonists in patients with decompensated heart failure. The same is true of ACE inhibition acutely, although this drug should be initiated once the patient is haemodynamically stable.

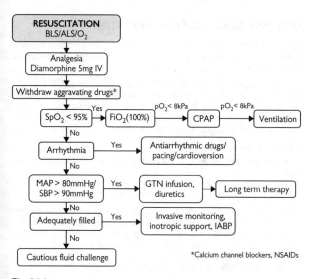

Fig. 24.1 Algorithm for the management of AHF. Reproduced from Myerson SG et al. *Emergencies in Cardiology*, 2005, (□ p. 73) with permission from Oxford University Press.

Oxygen and ventilatory support

Patients should initially receive 100% oxygen via a non-rebreathing face-mask. The maintenance of SaO_2 within the normal range is important to maximize tissue oxygenation.

For those patients who remain hypoxic, or have a rising pCO_2, ventilatory support should be considered. In the first instance, non-invasive ventilation can be used. If the patient has contra-indications to non-invasive ventilation or deteriorates despite it, then tracheal intubation and mechanical ventilation should be considered.

Non-invasive ventilation

There are two techniques that are possible options for the management of AHF:
- Continuous positive airways pressure (CPAP).
- Non-invasive positive pressure ventilation (NIPPV).

CPAP uses a tight fitting mask and valve to deliver high-flow oxygen. CPAP achieves pulmonary recruitment, and is associated with an increase in functional residual capacity. The improved pulmonary compliance, reduced transdiaphragmatic pressure swings, and decreased diaphragmatic activity can lead to a decrease in the overall work of breathing, and therefore a decreased metabolic demand from the body.

NIPPV is a more sophisticated technique that requires a ventilator. Addition of a PEEP to the inspiratory assistance results in a CPAP mode (also known as bi-level positive pressure support, BiPAP). The physiological benefits of this mode of ventilation are the same as for CPAP, but also include the inspiratory assist that further reduces the work of breathing and the overall metabolic demand.

CPAP and NIPPV decrease the need for endotracheal intubation, but there is no evidence that this translates into a reduction in mortality or improvement in long-term function.

Invasive mechanical ventilation

Invasive ventilation is indicated where the patient's airway is compromised by reduced conscious level (most commonly due to fatigue) or where there are contra-indications to non-invasive ventilation, including facial trauma. Respiratory fatigue manifests as a decrease in respiratory rate, with a rising pCO_2 and confusion.

Invasive mechanical ventilation can be used to facilitate immediate intervention in a patient with pulmonary oedema and ST-elevation myocardial infarction.

Key reference

Collins SP *et al.* The use of noninvasive ventilation in emergency department patients with acute cardiogenic pulmonary edema: a systematic review. *Ann Emerg Med* 2006; **48**: 260–9.

Pharmacological therapy

Opiates

Intravenous morphine/diamorphine reduces anxiety, as well as the effort of breathing. Morphine induces venodilatation and mild arterial dilatation, and reduces heart rate by an indirect reduction in sympathetic activity. These features reduce both pre-load and after-load.

An initial dose of 5mg morphine IV (2.5mg diamorphine IV) should be given and repeated as necessary, along with an anti-emetic.

Vasodilator therapy (📖 Chapter 37)

Vasodilators are currently considered the first-line therapy in the management of AHF by their reduction in both pre-load and after-load. The vasodilators most commonly used in AHF are nitrates, although sodium nitroprusside and nesiritide are also used.

1. Nitrates exert their effects in a dose-dependent fashion: at low doses they reduce pre-load by venodilatation, then as the dose is increased there is the additional effect of reduced afterload by arterial dilation. There is evidence that the combination of nitrates and furosemide is superior to high-dose diuretic treatment alone in the management of AHF. It has also been reported that intravenous high-dose nitrate is more effective than furosemide treatment in severe pulmonary oedema. Caution is required in patients with aortic stenosis.

Nitrates should be administered with careful BP monitoring. The dose should be reduced if systolic blood pressure falls below 90mmHg, and discontinued permanently if blood pressure drops further.
- s/l   2 puffs (400µg) of glyceryl trinitrate every 5 minutes
- buccal 1–5mg of isosorbide dinitrate
- IV   GTN 20–200µg/minute or isosorbide dinitrate 1–10mg/hour

2. Sodium nitroprusside is recommended for patients who require a predominant reduction in after-load (for example, hypertensive crisis, acute aortic or mitral regurgitation, or acute VSD). The dose should be titrated cautiously with invasive arterial monitoring. Prolonged administration may be associated with toxicity from its metabolites, thiocyanide and cyanide, and should be avoided especially in patients with severe renal or hepatic failure. As this drug is photosensitive, it requires careful preparation.

Administration: Initially 0.3µg/kg/minute uptitrating slowly to 10µg/kg/minute.

3. Nesiritide is a recombinant BNP that has venous, arterial, and coronary vasodilatory properties which reduce pre-load and after-load, and increase cardiac output without direct inotropic effects. But it is yet to be licensed in several countries, including the UK.

Diuretics (📖 Chapter 35)

Diuretics are indicated in patients with decompensated heart failure in the presence of fluid retention. They act by enhancing the excretion of water and sodium, leading to a decrease in plasma and extracellular fluid volume. Intravenous loop diuretics also exert an early venodilating effect, prior to their diuretic action. This manifests as a reduction in pre-load. Diuretics should be avoided in the acute setting if the systolic BP is <90mmHg.

Intravenous loop diuretics (furosemide, bumetanide, torasemide) should be given as a bolus, followed by a continuous infusion where necessary. The addition of a thiazide can augment diuresis and avoid the use of higher doses of a single drug, and its subsequent side-effects. The combination of loop diuretics with dopamine or nitrates is an alternative therapeutic approach.

Currently, there are a number of new agents with diuretic and additional effects that are under investigation, including the vasopressin V_2 receptor antagonist Tolvaptan, and the adenosine receptor antagonist, KW-3902.

Anticoagulation

Patients with AHF are at risk of venous thromboembolism, and should therefore be commenced on a low molecular weight heparin, for example, s/c enoxaparin 40mg/day if renal function is normal (otherwise 20mg/day).

Digoxin

In CHF, cardiac glycosides reduce hospitalizations by their effects on symptoms. In contrast, in AHF, cardiac glycosides produce a small increase in cardiac output and a reduction of filling pressures. However, digoxin is not indicated as an inotrope in AHF because of an associated increase in life-threatening arrhythmias. It is therefore paradoxical that the main indication for digoxin in AHF is to control the heart rate in tachyarrhythmias.

Inotropic agents and vasopressors (📖 Chapter 36)

Inotropic agents can be considered in patients who, despite diuretics and vasodilators at optimal tolerated doses, have peripheral hypoperfusion with hypotension and decreased renal function, ± pulmonary oedema.

As discussed in (📖 Chapter 36), there are significant detrimental effects of inotropes including
• Increased myocardial oxygen demand.
• Altered calcium loading.

These effects may exacerbate the heart failure syndrome or be pro-arrhythmic.

There are few controlled trials with inotropic agents in patients with AHF, and very few have assessed their effects on the symptoms and signs of heart failure and their long-term effects on prognosis.

In AHF, the inotropes most frequently used are **dopamine** and **dobutamine**. Tachycardia may be the limiting factor in the uptitration of these agents. In the presence of hibernating myocardium, dobutamine appears to achieve short-term increased contractility, but at the expense of myocyte necrosis.

The phosphodiesterase inhibitors (for example, **milrinone** and **enoximone**) are used to treat AHF in specific settings, including post-operative care of cardiac surgical patients.

Levosimendan was hoped to be the solution in inotropic therapy by achieving positive inotropic effect without calcium overload. It is a calcium-sensitizing agent that promotes inotropy by stabilizing troponin C in a configuration which enhances the calcium sensitivity of cardiac myofilaments. Unfortunately, trials to date have been disappointing. Levosimendan is not currently licensed for use in the UK or USA.

Vasopressors are indicated in AHF when the patient has an optimal filling pressure (CVP 10–14cmH$_2$O or PCWP 14–16mmHg), and the addition of an inotropic agent fails to restore adequate organ perfusion. Caution should be applied as the use of vasopressors may increase the afterl-oad and further reduce end-organ perfusion.

▶ In acute decompensated heart failure with significant renal dysfunction or hypotension, anti-RAAS therapy may need to be temporarily stopped.

Non-pharmacological therapy

Intra-aortic balloon pump (📖 Chapter 28)
An intra-aortic balloon pump (IABP) can be used to improve coronary artery perfusion and provide haemodynamic support in AHF where initial treatment options have been unsuccessful, and either a definitive treatment is planned or recovery is anticipated. Indications include
● Acute ischaemic cardiomyopathy.
● Cardiogenic shock post-MI.
● Fulminant myocarditis.
● Post-MI VSD.
● Post-MI mitral regurgitation (for example, papillary muscle infarction).

Ventricular assist devices
Until recently, cardiac assist devices (📖 Chapter 6) have required implantation in specialist cardiothoracic centres. However, lately, percutaneous devices have become available, although they are still to be subject to major trial. These temporary devices are potentially useful in bridging patients with AHF to stability/definite therapy, while avoiding some of the risks of a major surgical procedure.

Cardiac transplantation (📖 Chapter 9)
Urgent cardiac transplantation should be considered in patients with cardiogenic shock secondary to fulminant myocarditis or post-myocardial infarction where the prognosis would otherwise be poor.

Developing device therapies
The Tandem Heart™ is a continuous-flow centrifugal assist device, which is an attractive development in technology. A venous catheter is inserted via the femoral vein, and sits in the left atrium via a trans-septal puncture. Oxygenated blood is pumped out of the left atrium and propelled by the pump back into an arterial catheter inserted into the femoral artery. It is capable of flow rates up to 4L/minute. It has been shown to be beneficial

in stabilizing patients in cardiogenic shock in AMI to recovery or surgical intervention. However, there are concerns regarding severe bleeding and leg ischaemia.

Extracorporeal membrane oxygenation (ECMO) uses cardiopulmonary bypass technology to provide prolonged cardiac or respiratory support. ECMO is now an accepted practice for respiratory and/or cardiac failure in neonates, but its use in adults and children remains controversial.

Ultrafiltration is not a new concept in AHF. However, a portable machine has now been developed with peripheral IV catheters, offering the potential for use of this technique outside of intensive care or dialysis units. The RAPID-CHF trial peripheral veno-venous ultrafiltration (UF) was carried out in 40 hospitalized patients with AHF. Randomization was to 8 hours of UF + usual care versus usual care. The end-point of fluid removal at 24 hours (in millilitre) was significantly greater in the UF group.

Key reference

Bart BA *et al.* Ultrafiltration versus usual care for hospitalized patients with heart failure: the Relief for Acutely Fluid-Overloaded Patients With Decompensated Congestive Heart Failure (RAPID-CHF) trial. *J Am Coll Cardiol* 2005; **46**: 2043–6.

Management of specific AHF syndromes

Acute ischaemic cardiomyopathy

The key pathological process is ischaemia, and hence urgent coronary angiography with the ability of follow-on intervention should be considered. The patient may need to be stabilized to facilitate the procedure by means of an intra-aortic balloon pump and/or assisted ventilation. In some patients, there may be a role for mechanical LV support with an assist device and/or cardiac transplantation.

▶ Seek early involvement of an interventional cardiologist ± intensivist.

Valvular heart disease

AHF can be secondary to valvular conditions including
- Acute mitral valve incompetence.
- Acute aortic valve incompetence (including aortic dissection).
- Aortic stenosis.
- Mitral stenosis.
- Thrombosis of a prosthetic valve.
- Endocarditis.

In endocarditis, initial management of the haemodynamically stable patient is conservative therapy with antibiotic therapy. However, urgent surgery is indicated in patients with endocarditis and severe acute aortic regurgitation.

AHF from prosthetic valve thrombosis is associated with a high mortality (between 8 and 20%). If valve thrombosis is suspected and there is evidence of AHF, then the patient should be examined with fluoroscopy and echocardiography (TTE ± TOE). Thrombolysis is associated with a risk of embolization of thrombotic material. This may cause pulmonary embolism from right-sided valves, or potentially cause cerebrovascular events from left-sided valves. These risks are in addition to the 'usual' risks of haemorrhage. Thrombolysis is used for right-sided prosthetic valves, and for high-risk surgical candidates. Surgery should be discussed for left-sided prosthetic valve thrombosis, but thrombolysis may be the initial treatment of choice.

The thrombolytics used are:
- rtPA 10-mg IV bolus followed by 90mg infused over 90 minute.
- Streptokinase 250 000–500 000 U over 20 minute followed by 1–1.5 million U infused over 10 hours.

After completion of thrombolysis, unfractionated heparin should be administered by intravenous infusion in all patients (APTT ratio 1.5–2.0 times control).

AHF syndromes requiring surgical intervention
- Ventricular dysfunction.
  - Cardiogenic shock post-MI if PCI not feasible.
  - Post-MI ventricular septal rupture.
  - Ventricular free wall rupture.
- Valve disease.
  - Acute valve dysfunction.
  - Papillary muscle rupture.
  - Prosthetic valve failure or thrombosis.
- Aortic root disease:
  - Type A aortic dissection.
  - Ruptured aneurysm of sinus of Valsalva.

Cardiogenic shock and AMI

Cardiogenic shock is defined as the presence of all of the following:
- Systolic BP <90mmHg persisting for >30minutes.
- Elevated ventricular filling pressures (PCWP >18mmHg).
- Low cardiac output.
- End-organ hypoperfusion.

Cardiogenic shock is estimated to complicate 6–7% of AMI, usually involving ST-elevation MI, but non-ST-elevation acute coronary syndromes may also be the cause. The majority of cases (approximately 80%) result from severe left ventricular systolic dysfunction, while others have a mechanical defect (for example, acute VSD, acute RV infarction, or acute papillary muscle rupture). In-hospital mortality remains high at between 56% and 74%, irrespective of the presence or absence of ST elevation.

The patient with cardiogenic shock in the context of AMI needs to be recognized early and managed aggressively if appropriate to their comorbid condition. This includes
- Early echocardiogram to establish the aetiology of the shock.
- Invasive monitoring to facilitate optimization of BP and filling pressures.
    - Arterial cannula.
    - Central venous line ± pulmonary artery catheter.
- Inotropic support.
- Early use of an IABP.
- Referral for the consideration of emergency revascularization.

The 2005 ACC/AHA guidelines for PCI clearly advocate a role for primary PCI in these patients. Discussion with the local interventional centre should take place before thrombolysis is given. PCI should aim to maximally revascularize the patient: this is in contrast to PCI for AMI without shock where guidelines support infarct-related vessel revascularization only. If coronary angiography is not favourable for PCI, then emergency CABG should be considered. Alternative strategies include the use of LVADs or emergency cardiac transplantation.

The role of PCI and CABG in AMI have been discussed earlier. Cardiac surgery may also be indicated if the AHF results from:
- Acute valvular dysfunction.
- Acute ventricular septal/free wall rupture.
- Aortic dissection.

Predictors of mortality in AHF and AMI include

- Increasing age.
- Previous MI.
- Poor peripheral perfusion at presentation (cold, clammy, and confused).
- Oliguria.
- Delay in pain-to-reperfusion therapy.
- Severe LVSD at baseline echo.
- Moderate or severe mitral regurgitation at baseline echo.

Key trial[1, 2]

SHOCK—early revascularization in acute myocardial infarction complicated by cardiogenic shock. SHOCK Investigators. SHould We Emergently Revascularize Occluded Coronaries for Cardiogenic ShocK.

The SHOCK trial included 302 patients with cardiogenic shock within 36 hours of an AMI. They were randomized to emergency revascularization (36% CABG, 64% PCI) or medical stabilization. At 30 days there was no difference in outcome. At 6 months and beyond, there was a statistically significant increased survival in the group that underwent early revascularization.

Design: RCT of revascularization (36% CABG, 64% PCI) versus initial medical stabilization

Subjects: n = 302; NYHA IV; LVEF ≤35%; mean age = 65.8 years; 68% ♂; 60% anterior STEMI; median time MI to shock 5.6 hours

Follow-up: initially 6 months (latest update at 6 years)

Results: 30 days: 9.3% absolute difference in total mortality (47% revascularization versus 56% medical)

1 year: 13% absolute difference in total mortality

3 years: 13.1% absolute difference in total mortality

6 years: 13.12% absolute difference in total mortality (33% revascularization versus 20% medical)

1. Hochman JS et al. Early revascularization in acute myocardial infarction complicated by cardiogenic shock. SHOCK Investigators. SHould we emergently revascularize Occluded Coronaries for cardiogenic shocK. *N Engl J Med* 1999; **341**: 625–34.

2. Hochman JS et al. Early revascularization and long-term survival in cardiogenic shock complicating acute myocardial infarction. *JAMA* 2006; **295**: 2511–15.

Flash pulmonary oedema

Flash pulmonary oedema is the rapid development of symptoms and signs of AHF attributable to a number of conditions:

- Myocardial ischemia.
- Acute aortic incompetence.
- Acute mitral regurgitation.
- Critical mitral stenosis.
- Malignant hypertension (for example, secondary to phaeochromocytoma).
- Renal artery stenosis.
- Acute arrhythmia.

Flash pulmonary oedema is often associated with preserved systolic function. The differential diagnosis is:

- Pulmonary embolism.
- Pneumonia.
- Acute respiratory distress syndrome.

Specific investigation and management

Malignant hypertension is characterized by:

- Persistent diastolic BP >130mmHg.
- Fundal changes: retinal haemorrhages, exudates, and papilloedema.
- CNS—headache, confusion, seizures, and coma.
- Renal—oliguria and uraemia.

Patients with AHF due to hypertensive crisis require management in a high-dependency/intensive care setting with invasive arterial monitoring. Pharmacological therapy includes

- Diuretics, for example, IV furosemide 50–80mg bolus ± infusion of 10mg/hour. It is not recommended to exceed 4mg/minute except in single doses of up to 80mg.
- Vasodilators with nitrate moieties, for example, IV GTN 0.5–10mg/hour.
- Adrenergic agents, for example, IV labetalol 2mg/minute infusion.

Renal artery stenosis—recurrent episodes of flash pulmonary oedema in a patient with marked hypertension is an indication for the evaluation for renovascular disease; revascularization by percutaneous angioplasty should be considered if there is a ≥75% stenosis in one or both renal arteries.

Arrhythmias and AHF

Arrhythmias are common in AHF. These can be either supraventricular (in particular atrial fibrillation) or ventricular. They may be a cause or consequence of AHF, and can be life-threatening.

Bradycardias

Bradycardia in AHF patients occurs commonly in inferior myocardial infarctions, usually as a result of right coronary artery occlusion. The other frequent cause is iatrogenic from drug therapies, such as digoxin and β-adrenoreceptor antagonists.

The management of haemodynamically significant bradycardia secondary to AMI is initially atropine (and isoproterenol if necessary/available), or with the early consideration of temporary pacing in the face of AHF. Digoxin-induced bradycardia should be managed similarly with the withdrawal of digoxin. Rarely, Digibind™ may be required in cases of profound digoxin toxicity. In bradycardia secondary to β-adrenoreceptor antagonists, caution should be employed in stopping this therapy. Rather, the dose should be reduced in the first instance, where possible. However, glucagon can be used in cases of severe β-adrenoreceptor antagonist toxicity, unresponsive to atropine. The dose of glucagon is 2–10μg in 5% glucose followed by an IV infusion of 50μg/kg/hr.

Supraventricular tachycardia

Tachycardias are often poorly tolerated in patients with AHF, due to the reduction in ventricular filling time. Therefore, the control of the ventricular rate response is important. If haemodynamically compromised, this may be achieved with electrical cardioversion. If haemodynamics allows, then pharmacological cardioversion or rate control should be attempted.

It is important to ensure that patients with haemodynamically stable SVT are anticoagulated prior to cardioversion, unless the duration is <48 hours. The first-line drug of choice in the case of recent onset/anticoagulated is amiodarone; otherwise rate control can be achieved with digoxin.

▶ The introduction of β-adrenoreceptor antagonists in decompensated HF is not advised.

Ventricular tachycardia/fibrillation

Ventricular fibrillation and pulseless ventricular tachycardia require immediate cardioversion. Haemodynamically tolerated ventricular tachycardia should initially be treated with intravenous amiodarone. Individuals who do not respond to amiodarone therapy should be considered for overdrive pacing, which allows the option of suppression pacing thereafter, or a synchronized shock under sedation/general anaesthetic.

Discharge planning

After stabilization of AHF, steps should be taken to initiate a discharge plan. The patient should be free of dyspnoea and clinically euvolaemic. They should be at their dry weight, on oral diuretics with stable renal function, and off intravenous inotropic support for at least 48 hours.

Patients should be initiated on appropriate disease-modifying therapy, and arrangements made for review and uptitration within the following 1–2 weeks. Patients should also be able to mobilize around the ward, and complete basic activities of daily living.

Prior to discharge, time should be invested to educate the patient and their family regarding:
• The heart failure syndrome.
• Fluid and salt restriction.
• Monitoring of daily weights.
• Medication.
• Exercise.

Patients should also be empowered to recognize clinical deterioration and appreciate when to call for help. This can be facilitated by involvement of heart failure liaison nurses.

Section IV

Procedures

Central venous cannulation

Introduction

Central venous access is a key skill in the management of an ill patient. The Seldinger technique allows line placement into a variety of locations including veins, arteries, or the pleural cavity.

Indications for central vein cannulation include:
- Invasive pressure measurement.
- Pulmonary artery catheterization.
- Infusion of vasopressors.

The location of a central venous catheter can be:
- Internal jugular vein.
- Subclavian vein.
- Femoral vein.

The internal jugular vein is most often used as, compared to the femoral site, the site can be kept sterile. The internal jugular vein allows the catheter to be inserted under direct ultrasound guidance, thus reducing the potential for complications such as carotid artery puncture or pneumothorax.

Potential complications of central venous cannulation include:
- Bleeding.
- Vascular damage including late vessel stenosis.
- Arterial puncture.
- Pneumothorax (↑ risk with subclavian vein, not with femoral vein!).
- Infection (↑ with femoral vein, ↓ subclavian vein).
- Arrhythmia.
- Air embolism.

▶ NICE guidance from 2002 advised that ultrasound guidance should be used for the placement of all central venous catheters.

The technique (Fig. 25.1)
A critical aspect to any invasive procedure is scrupulous attention to aseptic technique. The skin should be prepared and draped after choosing the site of approach. Local anaesthetic should be infiltrated into the skin and subcutaneous tissues. The catheter is flushed in preparation for insertion. The patient is positioned supine ± head down tilt.
- An incision is made in the skin, then a needle is inserted into the vein.
- A J-tipped wire is advanced through the needle into the vein.
- The needle is removed leaving the wire in place.
- The skin is dilated with the dilator.
- The catheter can then be gently twisted into position.
- The guidewire is then removed.
- The catheter is sutured and the site covered with a sterile dressing.
- A check CXR should be performed except for femoral venous lines.

▶▶ Never advance the wire against resistance.

▶▶ Always ensure you have control and sight of the guidewire.

❶ Consider anatomy before cannulation in adult congenital heart disease.

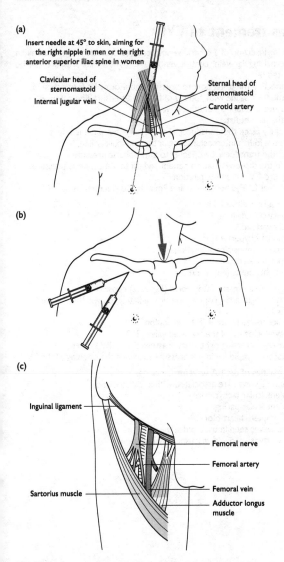

(a)

Insert needle at 45° to skin, aiming for
the right nipple in men or the right
anterior superior iliac spine in women

Clavicular head of
sternomastoid

Internal jugular vein

Sternal head of
sternomastoid

Carotid artery

(b)

(c)

Inguinal ligament

Sartorius muscle

Femoral nerve

Femoral artery

Femoral vein

Adductor longus
muscle

Fig. 25.1 (a) Anatomy of IJV. (b) Anatomy of subclavian vein. (c) Anatomy of femoral vein. Reproduced from Myerson SG *Emergencies in Cardiology*, 2005, (📖 pp. 291–293) with permission from Oxford University Press.

Measurement of CVP

Following insertion of a central venous catheter into either the subclavian or internal jugular vein, central venous (i.e. right atrial) pressure can be calculated by:
- Connecting the distal port to pressure-monitoring kit (consisting of 500mL 0.9% saline with 1000 U of heparin to ensure line patency, pressure transducer, and three-way tap).
- Lie the patient flat.
- Carefully place the transducer at the level of the patient's right atrium—fourth intercostal space in the mid-axillary line.
- Zero the transducer by opening to atmospheric pressure.
- Open the three-way tap to patient and off to atmospheric pressure.
- Measure CVP at end-expiration.
- A normal CVP is between 0 and 7mmHg (10–15cmH$_2$O).

RA pressure is elevated in:
- RV infarction/failure.
- Fluid overload.
- Pulmonary hypertension.
- Tricuspid stenosis/regurgitation.
- Pulmonary stenosis.
- Left–right shunts (e.g. VSD).

The right atrial pressure waveform (Fig. 25.2) consists of:
- **a wave**—right atrial contraction (immediately follows the P wave on ECG).
- **x descent**—right atrial (RA) relaxation.
- **c wave**—closure of the tricuspid valve (TV).
- **v wave**—increasing right atrial pressure during RV systole.
- **y descent**—rapid fall in RA pressure following the opening of the TV.

Abnormalities of the RA waveform include:
- Cannon a waves are associated with a–v dissociation.
  - Ventricular tachycardia.
  - Ventricular pacing.
  - Complete heart block.
- Tall a waves seen in tricuspid stenosis.
- Tall v waves seen with tricuspid regurgitation.

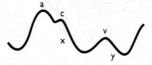

Fig. 25.2 The right atrial pressure waveform.

Cardiac catheterization

Introduction

Cardiac catheterization is invasive, and hence has the potential to cause the patient harm. However, despite advances in non-invasive imaging, there are frequent occasions when invasive investigation is required. Both right and left heart catheterization can offer valuable information about the patient.

Details of coronary angiography are not included, as this is the subject of entire books. It is a very important aspect of the assessment of heart failure. Coronary angiography is often performed prior to left ventricular assessment.

Pulmonary artery catheters

Pulmonary artery flotation catheters (PACs) are used to measure pressures in the right heart (right atrium, right ventricle, pulmonary artery, and pulmonary capillary wedge pressure), cardiac output (using thermodilution), pulmonary and systemic vascular resistance. They can also be used to detect intracardiac shunts (for example, ventricular septal defects).

The Swan–Ganz catheter for the measurement of cardiac output has four ports: balloon tip, proximal port, distal port that sits in the PA, and a thermistor that is located at the distal end of the catheter. The basic PAC has a balloon for flotation and a single lumen at the catheter tip. These catheters are ideally suited to be floated from the neck, rather than the femoral route.

Indications
- Cardiogenic shock.
- Pulmonary oedema.
- Right ventricular infarction.
- Shock of uncertain aetiology.
- Post-operative management of cardiac surgical patients.
- Massive pulmonary thromboembolism.
- Established LV systolic dysfunction with sepsis, acute hypovolaemia or during peri-operative care.
- Cardiac transplantation assessment.

Trials to study the benefits of PACs have been difficult to perform because of the extreme heterogeneity of the patient population. Two recent multi-centre prospective trials have been published, which may radically reduce the use of PACs:
- In an intensive care population that included patients with acute myocardial infarction, the FACTT trial concluded that PACs did not improve survival or organ function but were associated with more catheter-related complications, mainly arrhythmias.
- The ESCAPE trial looked specifically at the use of pulmonary artery catheters in guiding the management of patients with decompensated chronic heart failure, and concluded that there was no indication for the routine use of PACs.

PACs should be reserved for the patients being assessed for cardiac transplantation, those in whom there is clinical uncertainty as to their haemodynamic status (for example, right ventricular infarction), and those with established LV dysfunction and acute change in fluid status, for example, bleeding, sepsis, or renal failure.

The optimal filling pressure (PCWP) in the presence of LV systolic dysfunction is 14mmHg.

Key references

Wheeler AP *et al.* Pulmonary artery versus central venous catheter to guide treatment of acute lung injury. *N Engl J Med* 2006; **354**: 2213–24.
Binanay C *et al.* Evaluation study of congestive heart failure and pulmonary artery catheterization effectiveness: the ESCAPE trial. *JAMA* 2005; **294**: 1625–33.

Complications of PACs
- Complications of central venous cannulation.
- Arrhythmias—predominantly ventricular.
- Pulmonary haemorrhage.
- Pulmonary artery rupture.
- Pulmonary infarction.
- Valvular trauma—either tricuspid or pulmonary.
- Infection—potentially endocarditis.

Cautions
- Coagulopathy.
- Tricuspid valve disease—contra-indicated in prosthetic tricuspid valve replacement.

Technique
The catheter is most easily manipulated through the superior vena cava from the internal jugular vein or the subclavian vein, but can be introduced through the inferior vena cava from the femoral vein.

The potential for ventricular arrhythmias, particularly on crossing the tricuspid valve, requires that full resuscitation equipment should be available during manipulation of the PAC. Fluoroscopy should be used to place the PAC.

1. Ensure that IV access is patent, and that ECG monitoring is connected.
2. Insert a central venous introducer sheath into the central vein.
3. Flush all the lumens of the catheter and test the balloon with 1.6mL of air.
4. Connect the pressure line, with the transducer zeroed at the level of the right atrium, to the distal port of the PAC.
5. Insert the catheter 15cm, then inflate the balloon to assist with transit through the right heart.
6. Advance the catheter—the RV is usually entered with a catheter length of 25–35cm and the PA at 40–50cm. Aim for the pulmonary artery serving the lower third of the lung. Record the waveforms in the RA, RV, and PA (Fig. 26.1). When the PCWP trace appears, stop advancing the catheter and deflate the balloon. If the PA trace does not appear, withdraw the catheter by 2cm.
7. Gently re-inflate the balloon and measure the PCWP. A stable wedge position allows the catheter to be left in position with a PA trace that then shows a PCWP trace on balloon inflation. Measure PCWP at end-expiration (closest to atmospheric pressure).

▶▶ The balloon should not be left inflated because of the potential for trauma or pulmonary artery rupture.

▶▶ The balloon should not be inflated if resistance is felt.

Troubleshooting
Difficulty accessing the pulmonary artery or crossing the pulmonary valve

Try to torque the catheter anticlockwise after it crosses the tricuspid valve.

Ask the patient to take a deep breath in or cough once the catheter is through the tricuspid valve.

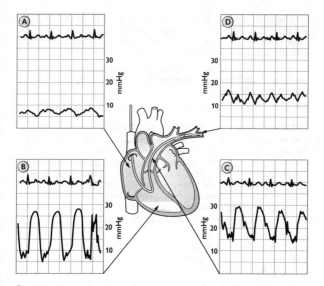

Fig. 26.1 Picture of waveforms. Reproduced from Myerson SG et al. *Emergencies in Cardiology*, 2005, (□ p. 295) with permission from Oxford University Press.

From the femoral route the catheter may point down into the right ventricular apex—force should not be applied to avoid perforation of the apex. If despite the above manoeuvres the tip does not point upwards, then a soft-tipped J-tipped wire (0.025 inch = 0.64mm diameter) may be introduced to steer the wire up into the right ventricular outflow tract.

Catheter knotting
- Try to prevent by avoiding excessive catheter loops.
- Do not pull the catheter tight.
- Ask for help.
- Try advancing the catheter and manipulating it with a guidewire.

If unable to untie the knot, do not pull back through the internal jugular veins. A snare may be used to retrieve the catheter through the femoral vein, or vascular surgery referral may be required.

Poor wedge trace
A good wedge trace has the left atrial waveform with 'a' and 'V' waves. PCWP cannot be higher than PA diastolic pressure. If the trace continues to rise on balloon inflation, it suggests 'over-wedging' and the balloon should be deflated and the catheter withdrawn by 2cm before re-inflation. If the trace appears damped, the catheter may be kinked.

If balloon inflation fails to alter the trace, the tip may have become displaced and requires re-manipulation, or the balloon may have ruptured requiring replacement of the catheter. Imaging the catheter tip with fluoroscopy may differentiate between these possibilities.

Severe mitral regurgitation results in a prominent systolic wave that may cause the PCWP trace to resemble the PA trace—measure PCWP at the end of the 'a' wave.

Remember that PCWP does not equal LVEDP in mitral stenosis.

Cardiac output measurement—thermodilution technique

This technique uses a modification of the Fick principle. A fixed volume (usually 10mL) of ice-cold saline is rapidly injected into the proximal port of the PAC. The rate of temperature change is detected by the thermistor at the catheter tip, 30cm distal. A cardiac output monitor needs to be set up with the volume of saline injected and the temperature. At least five measurements should be taken and averaged—more if atrial fibrillation or unstable rhythm. The readings should fall within 10% of each other and those with irregular traces should be discarded (Table 26.1).

Potential errors

- Valve lesions—tricuspid regurgitation allows some of the bolus to fall back into the RA; moderate or severe TR renders the technique meaningless.
- Septal defects.
- Leak in the connections.

Mixed venous oxygen saturation

Assuming that there is no intracardiac shunt, mixed venous oxygen saturation can be measured from a pulmonary artery blood sample—this should be taken slowly from the distal port to avoid 'arterialization', that is, pulmonary venous sampling. Normal mixed venous oxygen saturation is 70–75%. Low-output states result in increased tissue oxygen extraction, and so low mixed venous saturation. High mixed venous saturations occur in high-output states including septic shock, or in low-output states where there is a left-to-right shunt, for example, an acquired VSD.

Plasma lactate

In shock, tissue hypoxia prevents aerobic metabolism of pyruvate into water and carbon dioxide. Instead lactate is formed, and this can be measured offering useful data regarding tissue perfusion. A sample of either venous or arterial blood is collected into a heparin fluoride tube for analysis. Many arterial blood gas analyzers now measure lactate as standard. Normal plasma lactate is 0.3–1.3mmol/L. Initial rise in lactate may be seen after improving tissue perfusion, reflecting the washout from previously hypoperfused tissue.

Table 26.1 Interpretation of PAC data. (A-V SaO$_2$ is the difference in arterial and mixed venous oxygen saturations).

Normal values

Variable		Normal range
Stroke volume	SV	70–100mL
Cardiac output	CO	4–6L/minute
Right atrial pressure	RAP	0–5mmHg
Right ventricular pressure	RVP	20–25/0–5mmHg
Pulmonary artery pressure	PAP	20–25/10–15mmHg
Pulmonary capillary wedge pressure	PCWP	6–12mmHg
Mixed venous oxygen saturation	SVO$_2$	70–75%

Derived variables

Variable	Calculation	Normal range
Cardiac index (CI)	Cardiac output/BSA	2.5–3.5L/minute/m^2
Stroke index (SI)	Stroke volume/BSA	40–60mL/m^2
Systemic vascular resistance (SVR)	(MAP–RAP × 79.9)/CO	800–1400 dyne/s/cm^5
SVR Index	(MAP–RAP × 79.9)/CI	1760–2600 dyne/s/cm^5/m^2
Pulmonary vascular resistance	(PAP–PCWP × 79.9)/CO	25–125 dyne/s/cm^5

	Hypo-volaemia	Sepsis	LV failure	RV failure	Tamponade	Acquired VSD
CVP	↓	↓	↑	↑	↑	↑
PCWP	↓	↓	↑	↓	↑	↑
CO	↓	↑	↓	↓	↓	↓
SVR	↑	↓	↑	↑	↑	↑
A-V SaO$_2$	↑	↓	↑	↑	↑	↓

Reproduced from Grubb & Newby, *Churchills Pocketbook of Cardiology*, 2006, (📖 p. 61) with permission from Churchill Livingstone.

Measurement of left ventricular end diastolic pressure

The measurement of LVEDP contributes to the assessment of left ventricular filling pressures. The catheter is passed through the aortic valve from an arterial puncture as part of a left heart catheterization study. The traces can be recorded. The normal LVEDP is <12mmHg. The LVEDP can be elevated because of mitral incompetence, aortic incompetence, ventricular septal defect, or LV systolic dysfunction. The LVEDP can also be elevated if there is myocardial hypertrophy (for example, hypertensive heart disease) or myocardial infiltration (for example, amyloid) (Figs 26.2 and 26.3).

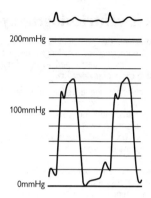

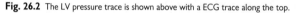

Fig. 26.2 The LV pressure trace is shown above with a ECG trace along the top.

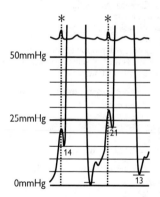

Fig. 26.3 This close-up view of the LVEDP has had the scale modified to ensure accurate measurement. The point to assess the LVEDP is indicated (*)—it is the point of the trace that equates to the peak of the R wave. The mean of several traces should be taken (3 if sinus rhythm, 5 if atrial fibrillation).

Contrast left ventriculography

This is considered to be the gold-standard assessment of LVEF. The quality of non-invasive imaging now challenges this position. It is invasive and is therefore infrequently performed as the routine follow-up for patients. It is useful in cases of uncertainty.

The procedure involves passing a pigtail catheter into the LV cavity. Often an angled pigtail is used to minimize the catheter entanglement in the mitral valve apparatus, and hence reduce ectopy. A power injector is then used to deliver contrast. Typical settings are 30–45mL of contrast at a rate of 10–15mL/second. The images are acquired in the following views (ideally with biplane imaging):

- 30° RAO projection.
  - Views high lateral, anterior, apical, and inferior walls.
- 45–60° LAO with 20° cranial tilt.
  - Views lateral and septal walls.
  - Best view to assess for VSD.

Indications for contrast left ventriculography

- Assessment of LVEF in patients with:
  - Ischaemic heart disease.
  - Valvular heart disease.
  - Cardiomyopathy.
- Assessment of regional wall motion abnormalities.
- Identification and assessment of ventricular septal defect.
- Assessment of mitral regurgitation.

Contra-indications to contrast left ventriculography

- Significant left main stenosis.
- Significant aortic valve stenosis.
- Renal impairment.
- LVEDP ≥25mmHg.
- LV systolic pressure ≥180mmHg.

Complications of contrast left ventriculography

- Cardiac arrhythmias.
- Intramyocardial staining.
- Embolism.
- Contrast reactions.

The images can be assessed after the procedure, and detailed measurements obtained of ventricular volumes, and hence LVEF, and regional wall motion. LVEF can be calculated from the following equation:

(end-diastolic volume–end-systolic volume)/end-diastolic volume × 100

The severity of mitral regurgitation is assessed from the degree of opacification of the left atrium during contrast left ventriculography as illustrated in 📖 Fig. 26.4.

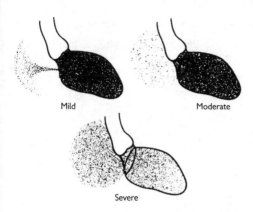

Fig. 26.4 Assessment of severity of mitral regurgitation from contrast left ventriculography. Reproduced from Figure 4–23 of Morton L Kern, *The Cardiac Catheterisation Handbook*, 2003, Mosby with permission from Elsevier.

Chapter 27

Endomyocardial biopsy

Introduction

In 1962, Sakakibara and Konno first reported their experience with transvascular cardiac biopsy (Fig. 27.1). In 1973, Caves *et al.* first described transvenous endomyocardial biopsy to diagnose cardiac allograft rejection.

There are few occasions when an endomyocardial biopsy is necessary in patients with chronic heart failure. Rare exceptions are where an infiltrative cardiac condition is suspected, although diagnostic information can often be obtained by other methods. In an acute presentation of new heart failure, endomyocardial biopsy is indicated if giant cell myocarditis is suspected.

Right ventricular endomyocardial biopsies are common practice following cardiac transplantation to identify the evidence of allograft rejection, being generally performed weekly for the first 6 weeks, then fortnightly to 3 months, and then every 6 weeks for the remainder of the first postoperative year. Only in very rare instances is a left ventricular biopsy indicated (e.g. due to multiple previous RV biopsies) due to the risk of systemic embolization.

Indications

Acute heart failure:
• Giant cell myocarditis.
• Hyper-eosinophilic myocarditis.

Chronic heart failure:
• Amyloidosis.
• Sarcoidosis.
• Haemochromatosis.
• ?Chagas.
• ?Fabry.

Post-cardiac transplantation.

Potential complications

Total procedural risk of approximately 1%.
• Arrhythmias.
• Tamponade.
• Pneumothorax.
• Conduction disturbance.
• Air embolism.
• Nerve palsy.

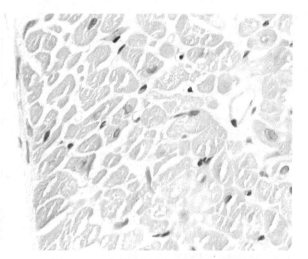

Fig. 27.1 (See colour plate 8) Normal endocardium and myocardium. The endocardium on the left is a thin uniform layer with underlying myocardium that comprises cardiac myocytes, which are closely applied to one another with little intervening stroma that includes small blood vessels. Haematoxylin and eosin ×400. Courtesy of Dr Allan McPhaden, Glasgow Royal Infirmary.

Procedure

Generally a right internal jugular approach is undertaken, although the femoral route can be employed with the use of a long venous sheath.

▶ Ask your pathologist beforehand:
- How many biopsy specimens are required?
- What are the samples should be fixed in?

- Insert 9F RIJ sheath with haemostasis valve (see 📖 Chapter 25).
- Before use, the bioptome must first be checked to ensure:
  - The jaws approximate tightly.
  - The 90° bend lines up with the bioptome handle to aid guidance.
- Ask the patient to stop breathing when putting the bioptome into the sheath (and again when removing).
- Using fluoroscopy, direct the bioptome laterally along the SVC.
- In the mid-RA, rotate the bioptome anteriorly through the tricuspid valve.
- Advance into the RV gradually rotating posteriorly to the RV apex.
- Withdraw the tip slightly when it abuts the endocardium (seen fluoroscopically and felt as slight resistance).
- Open the bioptome jaws.
- Advance again onto the endocardial surface.
- Close the jaws of the bioptome and withdraw briskly but smoothly.
- Gently remove tissue sample from the jaws and place in appropriate preservative.

For cardiac allograft rejection assessment:
- Four to six biopsy specimens are obtained from each procedure (due to the multi-focal nature of rejection).
- Biopsies are fixed in 10% neutral buffered formalin.

Grades of cellular rejection on endomyocardial biopsy (ISHLT scale) (Figs 27.2 and 27.3):
- 0—no rejection.
- Ia—focal infiltrate without necrosis.
- Ib—diffuse but sparse infiltrate but without necrosis.
- II—one focus only, with aggressive infiltration and/or focal myocyte damage.
- IIIa—multi-focal aggressive infiltrates and/or myocyte damage.
- IIIb—diffuse inflammatory process with necrosis.
- IV—diffuse aggressive polymorphous infiltrate, and/or oedema, and/or haemorrhage, and/or vasculitis, with necrosis.

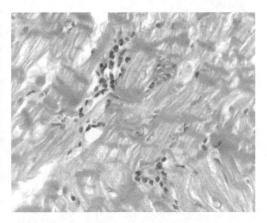

Fig. 27.2 (See colour plate 9) Low-grade cardiac allograft rejection. The myocardium contains small perivascular aggregates of mononuclear cells (ISHT Grade 1a). Haematoxylin and eosin ×400. Courtesy of Dr Allan McPhaden, Glasgow Royal Infirmary.

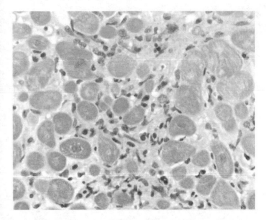

Fig. 27.3 (See colour plate 10) High-grade cardiac allograft rejection. The myocardium contains perivascular aggregates of mononuclear cells with extension into the interstitium associated with mutiple foci of cardiac myocyte degeneration. Haematoxylin and eosin ×400. Courtesy of Dr Allan McPhaden, Glasgow Royal Infirmary.

Chapter 28

IABP insertion

Introduction

An IABP comprises a 30–50mL, depending on the patient's height, helium-filled balloon placed in the descending thoracic aorta, connected to a pneumatic pump. The pump can be triggered from the ECG trace (or less commonly from the pressure trace) and inflates the balloon during diastole, and then rapidly deflates the balloon in systole. Balloon inflation augments diastolic blood pressure, resulting in improved coronary and cerebral perfusion. Balloon deflation reduces after-load and peripheral vascular resistance, and increases stroke volume. Unlike inotropes and vasopressors, the benefits of the balloon pump are not accompanied by an increase in myocardial oxygen demand.

Indications

An IABP can be used to improve coronary artery perfusion and/or provide haemodynamic support in cardiogenic shock of any cause.
- Acute coronary ischaemia resistant to pharmacological therapy ± ventricular arrhythmias ± cardiogenic shock (bridge to PCI or CABG).
- Cardiogenic shock.
- Post-operative in cardiac surgery.
- Acute VSD or mitral regurgitation post-MI.
- Prophylactic use for high-risk PCI or CABG.

Contra-indications

- Known aortic dissection.
- Abdominal aortic aneurysm.
- Significant aortic regurgitation.
- Patent ductus arteriosus.
- Severe peripheral vascular disease.

Complications

- Limb ischaemia (5–19%).
- Aortic dissection (<5%).
- Aorto-iliac perforation.
- Infection.
- Haemorrhage.

Insertion

IABP can be inserted using a femoral artery sheath; however, fewer vascular complications occur if a sheathless technique is adopted. The IABP comes in a box complete with the guidewire, pressure, and inflation lines. The size of balloon is determined by the patient's height correlated with the sizing chart on the IABP box.

- Prepare the inguinal region overlying the femoral artery for cannulation. Clean the skin down the medial aspect of the leg to the level of the knee. Drapes should cover a wide area to allow room to place the guidewire. Infiltrate the skin around the planned puncture site with local anaesthetic, ensuring adequate local anaesthesia around femoral artery.
- The Seldinger technique is used to cannulate the femoral artery, and then pass the guidewire up the aorta under fluoroscopic screening. The wire should be seen to sit in the aortic arch.
- For sheathless insertion, dilators are used to expand the skin and subcutaneous tissues before the IABP catheter is inserted over the wire into the femoral artery. Alternatively, the sheath provided is sited in the femoral artery and then the IABP catheter is placed.
- The tip of the IABP catheter should be advanced with fluoroscopic guidance until it sits below the left subclavian artery—no reduction in pulse character should be felt at the left radial artery.
- The catheter is then fixed in place with sutures both at the groin, and the shaft of the catheter is sutured to the medial aspect of the leg. The pressure lines and inflation lines should then be connected and the pump commenced.
- Systemic anticoagulation with intravenous heparin should be used to reduce the risk of arterial thrombosis. The IABP should not be switched off for more than 1 minute at a time to minimize the risk of thrombus formation.

Removal

The heparin infusion should be stopped, and the activated clotting time allowed to fall to <150 seconds. To reduce trauma at the femoral puncture site, the balloon inflation lines should be disconnected before pulling the catheter. As the IABP creates a sizeable hole in the femoral artery, the wound is best compressed with a mechanical clamp for at least 30 minutes.

IABP waveforms

Modern IABP pumps have detailed algorithms that optimize the timing of inflation and deflation of the balloon. ECG leads should be connected as inflation is usually triggered by the R wave. In certain situations, the pressure trace may be used to trigger the balloon. Usually the balloon inflates with each cardiac cycle (1:1 augmentation), but this can be reduced to 1:2 or 1:3 augmentation either to allow adequate filling time during tachycardias or to allow weaning of IABP support (Figs 28.1–28.5).

A patient with an IABP *in situ* requires close observation.

▶▶ If blood is noted in the inflation lines, this indicates that the balloon has ruptured. To prevent the balloon filling with blood and then clotting, the pump should be stopped and the balloon removed as soon as possible.

A = One complete cardiac cycle
B = Unassisted aortic end diastolic pressure
C = Unassisted systolic pressure
D = Diastolic augmentation
E = Reduced aortic end diastolic pressure
F = Reduced systolic pressure

Inflation Deflation

Fig. 28.1 Normal inflation/deflation cycle[*].

Inflation of the IAB prior to aortic calve closure

Waveform characteristics:
• Inflation of IAB prior to dicrotic notch.
• Diastolic augmentaion encroaches onto systole, (may be unable to distinguish).

Physiologic effects:
• Potential premature closure of the aortic value.
• Potential increase in LVEDV and LVEDP or PCWP.
• Increased left ventricular wall stress or afterload.
• Aortic regurgitation.
• Increased MVO_2 demand.

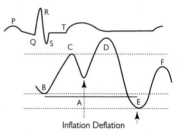

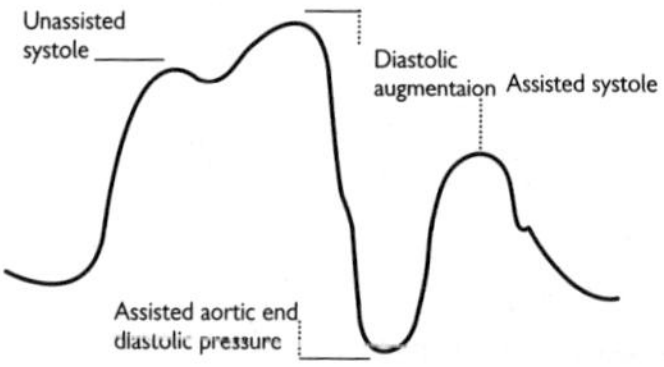

Unassisted systole

Diastolic augmentaion Assisted systole

Assisted aortic end diastulic pressure

Fig. 28.2 Early inflation of IABP[*].

Inflation of the IAB markedly after
closure of the aortic valve.

Waveform charcteristics:
• Inflation of IAB after the dicrotic notch.
• Absence of sharp V.

Physiologic effects:
• Sub-optimal coronary artery perfusion.

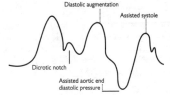

Fig. 28.3 Late inflation of IABP[*].

Premature deflation of the IAB during
the diastolic phase.

Waveform characteristics:
• Deflation of IAB is seen as a sharp
  drop following diastolic augmentation.
• Sub-optimal diastolic augmentation.
• Assisted aortic end diastolic pressure
  may be equal to or less than the
  unassisted aortic end diastolic pressure.
• Assisted systolic pressure may rise.

Physiologic effects:
• Sub-optimal coronary perfusion.
• Potential for retrograde coronary
  and carotid blood flow.
• Sub-optimal afer load reduction.
• Increased MVO_2 demand.

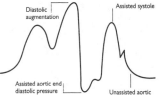

Fig. 28.4 Early deflation of IABP[*].

Waveform characteristics:
• Assisted aortic end diastolic pressure
  may be equal to the unassisted
  aortic end diastolic pressure.
• Rate of rise of assisted systole
  is prolonged.
• Diastolic augmentaion may appear
  widened.

Physiologic effects:
• Afterload reduction is essentially
  absent.
• Increased MVO_2 consumption due to
  the left ventricle ejecting against a
  greater resistance and a prolonged
  isovolumetric contraction phase.
• IAB may impede left ventricular
  ejection and increase the afterload.

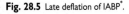

Fig. 28.5 Late deflation of IABP[*].

Cardiopulmonary exercise testing

Introduction

Cardiopulmonary exercise testing (CPET) is a non-invasive, dynamic study that provides an overall assessment of the physiological response to exercise. CPET is a better predictor of exercise performance and functional capacity than resting cardiac and pulmonary parameters. It has also been consistently related to morbidity and mortality.

Indications for CPET in CHF

Assessment of:
- Functional capacity (peak VO_2).
- Exercise-limiting symptoms.
- Breathlessness out-of-proportion to cardiac dysfunction.
- Prognosis.
- Selection for cardiac transplantation.

Measurements

The key measurements made during CPET include:
- VO_2 — respiratory oxygen uptake.
- VCO_2 — carbon dioxide production.
- RER — respiratory exchange ratio.
- Other ventilatory parameters:
  - Respiratory rate.
  - Tidal volume.
  - Minute ventilation (V_E).
  - Ventilatory threshold (V_T)—formerly known as anaerobic threshold—is the point at which V_E increases disproportionately to VO_2. It can be used to distinguish between cardiac and non-cardiac dyspnoea.
  - V_E/VCO_2.
  - Pulmonary gas exchange.
- Cardiac parameters including heart rate response.
- Borg scale rating of perceived dyspnoea.

Methodology

Patients undergoing CPET exercise on either a bicycle ergometer or treadmill. They wear a nose clip and breathe through a mouthpiece or a tightly fitting face mask. pO_2 and pCO_2 may be measured by a gas analyzer or pulse oximetry if the test is completely non-invasive. VO_2 and VCO_2 are calculated from the differences between inspired and expired gases and ventilatory volumes.

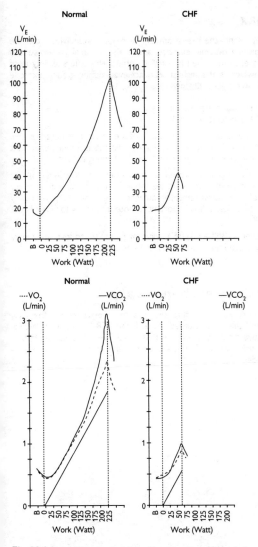

Fig. 29.1 Heart failure is associated with an increase in V_E due to increased dead space ventilation, to poor ventilation/perfusion matching, and a reduced workload and peak VO_2. Images courtesy of Dr Roger Carter, Glasgow Royal Infirmary.

VO$_2$ max

VO$_2$max represents the largest amount of oxygen an individual can use while performing dynamic exercise, and is the maximal arterio-venous oxygen difference multiplied by cardiac output. This differs slightly from peak VO$_2$, which is the highest VO$_2$ achieved during graded exercise testing. VO$_2$max is generally lower in:
- Women.
- Elderly individuals (declines with age).
- Those with a sedentary lifestyle.

VO$_2$max is often quoted as a percentage of predicted value based on age, sex, weight, and height. Some would argue that this is a more important prognostic marker than VO$_2$max, particularly in young patients.

In the presence of β-adrenoreceptor antagonism, a peak VO$_2$ ≤12mL/kg/ minutes should be used to guide the listing for transplantation. In those intolerant of a β-adrenoreceptor antagonist, a peak VO$_2$ ≤14mL/kg/ minute should be used. It is important to note that listing for CTx is not solely on VO$_2$.

In obese patients (BMI >30kg/m^2), adjusting peak VO$_2$ to lean body mass may be considered appropriate (using an adjusted cut-off of ≤19mL/kg/ minutes).

Respiratory exchange ratio

The respiratory exchange ratio (RER) is the ratio between the CO$_2$ produced and the O$_2$ consumed. At rest, the RER is around 0.70–0.85, but to achieve a maximal test the RER should be >1.05 indicating that CO$_2$ production exceeds O$_2$ uptake, and that the anaerobic threshold has been exceeded.

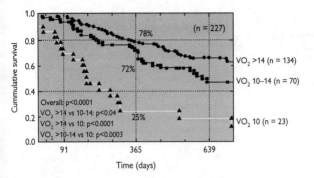

Fig. 29.2 Cumulative survival curves stratified by peak VO₂. Lund LH, Aaronson KD & Mancini DM. Validation of peak exercise oxygen consumption and the Heart Failure Survival Score for serial risk stratification in advanced heart failure. *Am J Cardiol* 2005; **95**: 734–41 with permission from Elsevier.

Chapter 30

Assessment of dyssynchrony

Introduction

With cardiac resynchronization therapy (CRT), at least 70% of patients improve symptomatically or demonstrate recovery in left ventricular systolic function. This is a more consistent and significant result than seen with any individual pharmacological agent. CRT improves symptoms, quality of life, and exercise tolerance. It also reduces mitral regurgitation.

Current recommendations for patient selection are based on the CARE-HF criteria including patients who, despite optimal tolerated medical therapy, have:
- NYHA class III with established severe LVSD.
- Ejection fraction ≤35%.
- Sinus rhythm.
- QRS duration >120ms.

However, those with QRS duration between 120 and 149ms were included in CARE-HF if there was evidence of dyssynchrony on transthoracic echocardiography. The CARE-HF study looked at three parameters to describe intraventricular dyssynchrony:
- Aortic pre-ejection time >140ms.
- Interventricular delay >40ms.
- Evidence of septal-to-lateral wall delay.

Electrical dyssynchrony as demonstrated by a prolongation in QRS duration does not always correlate with mechanical dyssynchrony. There is evidence that those individuals in whom there is significant dyssynchrony assessed by echocardiography at baseline benefit the most, and that benefit is as a result of the reduction in the level of dyssynchrony.

There are many different techniques to assess dyssynchrony including standard echo, tissue Doppler imaging, and contrast echo. Studies are ongoing that use tagged MRI to document dyssynchrony before device implantation. While many of these techniques offer improved imaging and document interventricular dyssynchrony, at present the evidence is based on the standard echo techniques used in CARE-HF. Additional details may be established from imaging, for example, the presence of infarct scar that may interfere with the LV epicardial pacing lead threshold.

The PROSPECT trial is aiming to identify the predictors of response to CRT. It completes recruiting in 2006, and is due to report in 2007, and will hopefully fill some of the gaps in the current understanding of CRT responders.

Assessment of intraventricular dyssynchrony

Measurement of aortic pre-excitation time[*]

APET is the interval between the onset of the QRS complex and the onset of aortic flow using pulsed wave Doppler.

Interventricular delay[*]

Interventricular delay is the interval between the onset of pulmonary ejection and aortic ejection using pulsed wave Doppler. A delay of >40ms is suggestive of significant intraventricular dyssynchrony.

Delayed activation of the posterolateral LV wall[*]

Defined as the maximal posterolateral wall inward movement, using M-mode or tissue Doppler imaging, occurring later than the start of LV filling, using the transmitral Doppler flow signal. Post-hoc analysis of the CARE-HF trial has suggested that this method of assessing dysynchrony is not very useful.

Alternatively, septal-to-posterior wall motion delay (SPWMD), using an M-mode recording from the parasternal short-axis view (at the level of the papillary muscles), can be obtained, and a cut-off value of ≥130ms was proposed as a marker of intraventricular dyssynchrony.

---

[*] See Leeson et al., *Echocardiography*, 2007 (p. 204), Oxford University Press.

Tissue Doppler imaging[*]

CARE-HF was the landmark trial that defined the role of CRT in CHF. The parameters described earlier were used to identify dyssynchrony in this trial. However, the method that is used most often in current clinical practice to assess dyssynchrony in CHF is tissue Doppler imaging (TDI). This method uses Doppler echo to measure the velocity of segments of left ventricular myocardial movement within the heart.

TDI can be performed using dedicated echo packages. There are a number of different techniques using samples from different segments of the LV (Figs. 30.1 and 30.2).

- The simplest method looks at the time from the beginning of the QRS complex on ECG to peak systolic velocities in the septum and lateral wall. The difference between the two peak systolic velocities was calculated as a measure of intraventricular dyssynchrony. This is described as the septal-to-lateral delay.
- A more complex method defines dyssynchrony from the maximum delay between the time from the beginning of the QRS complex on the ECG to peak systolic contraction velocity among four LV walls:
  - Anterior.
  - Inferior.
  - Septal.
  - Lateral.
- Perhaps, the most comprehensive use of TDI acquires from peak velocities in eight LV segments, four basal and four mid-left ventricular segments. Dyssynchrony is then defined by:
  - Maximum difference in time to peak contraction (Ts-diff).
  - Standard deviation in the time to peak contraction (Ts-SD).

Prolonged Ts-diff (>91ms) and Ts-SD (>37ms) were associated with a significant ↑ in all clinical events.

Ts-diff (>91ms) was an independent risk factor of clinical events and mortality, regardless of age, LVEF, QRSd, and use of β-adrenoreceptor antagonists.

Key references

Bax JJ et al. Left ventricular dyssynchrony predicts response and prognosis after cardiac resynchronisation therapy. J Am Coll Cardiol 2004; **44**: 1834–40.

Cho GY et al. Mechanical dyssynchrony assessed by tissue Doppler imaging is a powerful predictor of mortality in congestive heart failure with normal QRS duration. J Am Coll Cardiol 2005; **46**: 2237–43.

[*] See Leeson et al., Echocardiography, 2007 (p. 206), Oxford University Press.

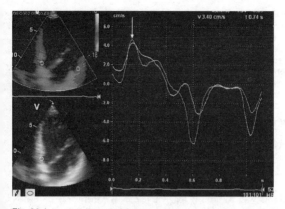

Fig. 30.1 (See colour plate 11) The assessment of LV dyssynchrony in a normal individual. In the colour-coded tissue Doppler images, sample volumes are placed in the basal part of the septum and lateral wall. Velocity graphs derived from the velocities measured in these sample volumes are presented. LV dyssynchrony is not present, as indicated by a septal-to-lateral delay in peak systolic velocity (↓) of 0ms. Reproduced from Westenberg JJM et al. Assessment of left ventricular dyssynchrony in patients with conduction delay and idiopathic dilated cardiomyopathy: head-to-head comparison between tissue doppler imaging and velocity-encoded magnetic resonance imaging. *J Am Coll Cardiol* 2006; **47**: 2042–8 with permission from Elsevier.

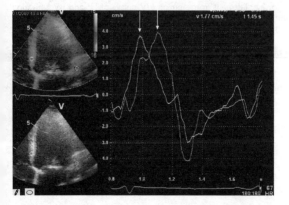

Fig. 30.2 (See colour plate 12) LV dyssynchrony assessment in CHF. There is extensive LV dyssynchrony with a septal-to-lateral delay in peak systolic velocities of 115ms (the time between the arrows).Reproduced from Westenberg JJM et al. Assessment of left ventricular dyssynchrony in patients with conduction delay and idiopathic dilated cardiomyopathy: head-to-head comparison between tissue doppler imaging and velocity-encoded magnetic resonance imaging. *J Am Coll Cardiol* 2006; **47**: 2042–8 with permission from Elsevier.

After CRT implantation, the device can be fine-tuned to optimize the effect on the left ventricular systolic function[*]. Some devices are incorporating technology that allows the CRT device to optimize itself without the need for echo studies. AV delays affect pre-excitation of the ventricles, and hence affect LV filling times:

• Short AV delay results in an earlier E-wave and a longer LV filling time, but because of early mitral valve closure reduces the left atrial contribution to LV filling.
• Long AV delay results in a delayed E-wave and shortens LV filling time.

AV delay optimization selects the shortest AV delay that avoids compromise of left atrial contributions to left ventricular filling. In the majority of patients, comparable mechanical benefits are achieved across a moderate range of AV delays, with optimal ventricular function at approximately:

$$((\text{Intrinsic PR duration}/2) - 30)\ \text{ms}.$$

Most patients have an acceptable result with an AV delay of 120ms. In patients with particularly long intrinsic delays, there may be benefit in testing a range of AV delays and selecting the optimal value for the individual.

'Dual chamber' (DDD) pacing, i.e. pacing of the atrium rather than simply sensing to facilitate AV timing, may be required if there is symptomatic bradycardia due to sinus node disease. This pacing mode will introduce intra-atrial conduction delay that alters the AV delay.

There is preliminary data suggesting that sequential biventricular pacing, rather than simultaneous, can improve systolic function. Pacing technology allows adjustment in the timing (VV delay) of LV and RV activation separately. Most patients benefit from slightly premature LV activation (Fig. 30.3).

[*] See Leeson *et al.*, *Echocardiography*, 2007 (p. 208), Oxford University Press.

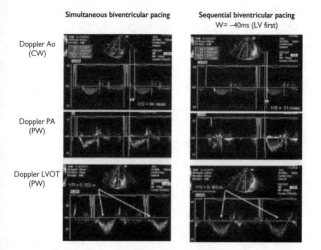

Fig. 30.3 Doppler echocardiography of the aorta (Ao), pulmonary artery (PA), and left ventricular outflow tract (LVOT) during simultaneous (left) and sequential biventricular pacing (right). Adjusting the VV delay to −40ms results in a higher LVOT velocity-time integral (VTI), together with less interventricular dyssynchrony as evidenced by the lower interventricular delay (IVD). CW = continuous wave; PW = pulsed wave; ↔ = interventricular delay (IVD). Reproduced from Vanderheyden M et al. Tailored echocardiographic interventricular delay programming further optimizes left ventricular performance after cardiac resynchronization therapy. *Heart Rhythm* 2005; **2**: 1066–72.

Key reference

Auricchio A et al. Effect of pacing chamber and atrioventricular delay on acute systolic function of paced patients with congestive heart failure. The Pacing Therapies for Congestive Heart Failure Study Group. The Guidant Congestive Heart Failure Research Group. *Circulation* 1999; **99**: 2993–3001.

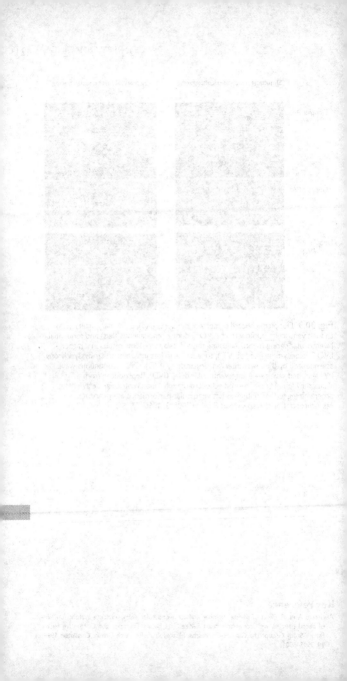

Section V

Detailed pharmacology and evidence base for drugs

ACE inhibitors

The renin–angiotensin–aldosterone system (RAAS)

ACE inhibitors were first introduced because of their vasodilatory properties. It is now understood that the beneficial effects arise from the antagonism of the RAAS (Fig. 31.1).

As has been mentioned in (📖 Chapter 2), increased RAAS activity causes deleterious effects on the cardiovascular system and contributes to the poor prognosis in CHF.

The next four chapters will demonstrate the rationale for the current pharmacological treatment for CHF is in the antagonism of the RAAS and sympathetic nervous systems.

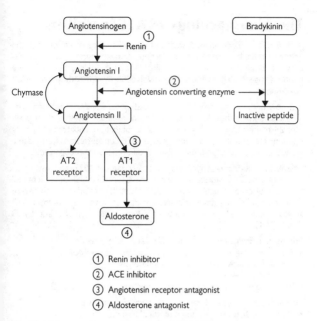

① Renin inhibitor
② ACE inhibitor
③ Angiotensin receptor antagonist
④ Aldosterone antagonist

Fig. 31.1 The sites of action of antagonists of the RAAS.

The pharmacology of ACE inhibitors

ACE is a zinc metallopeptidase found on the surface of endothelial and epithelial cells. It leads to the production of angiotensin II and the breakdown of bradykinin. The wide distribution and multiple actions of these peptides suggest that ACE could be involved in various pathophysiological conditions.

It is now understood that ACE concentrations are under genetic control. This was initially thought to be due to an insertion/deletion (I/D) polymorphism in intron 16; however, this is subject to debate and varying opinion. This translates to stable plasma ACE concentrations in the same individual, whereas large inter-individual differences are recognized.

The ACE inhibitor, captopril, was first described in 1977, and yet it was not until a decade had passed before the CONSENSUS study identified this class of drug to significantly reduce mortality in patients with severe CHF. ACE inhibitors have now become the cornerstone therapy for all stages of heart failure, as well as in patients with asymptomatic LVSD (Table 31.1).

Pharmacologically, there are three classes of ACE inhibitors:
- An active drug as well as active metabolites (e.g. captopril).
- A pro-drug, activated by hepatic metabolism
  (e.g. enalapril → enalaprilat).
- Water soluble and renally excreted unchanged (e.g. lisinopril).

Potential benefits of ACE inhibitors include reductions in:
- Myocardial hypertrophy and interstitial fibrosis.
- Atheroma.
- Oxidative stress.
- Fibrinogen.
- LV remodelling.

In CHF, this translates to:
- A reduction in morbidity.
- A reduction in mortality.
- An improvement in LVEF.

Table 31.1 The pharmokinetics of ACE inhibitors

ACE inhibitor	Zinc ligand	Pro-drug	Bio-availability (%)	Plasma protein binding (%)	Half-life (hours)	Excreted
Captopril	Sulphydril	No	60–75	30	2–3	Renal
Enalapril	Carboxyl	Yes	60*	50–60*	11	95% renal
Lisinopril	Carboxyl	No	6–60	Low	12	Renal
Perindopril†	Carboxyl	Yes	60	10–20	25–30	75% renal
Ramipril	Carboxyl	Yes	50–60*	56*	13–17	60% renal
Trandolapril†	Carboxyl	Yes	40–60*	80–94	16–24	33% renal

* Reflects the data of the active drug.
† No evidence in heart failure.

How to initiate (see also 📖 Chapter 5)

- Recommended in NYHA I–IV CHF and asymptomatic LVSD.
- Monitor blood pressure and renal function.
  - Aim for systolic BP >90mmHg.
- Double dose every 2–4 weeks if tolerated (could be increased more quickly following admission to hospital with acute heart failure, with adequate monitoring of blood pressure and renal function).
- Aim for target dose (see Table 31.2).

▶ A small dose is better than no dose at all!

Contra-indications to initiation

- Angio-oedema.
- Bilateral renal artery stenosis.
- Severe renal failure without renal replacement therapy.
- Hyperkalaemia.
- Pregnancy.
- The following are not absolute contra-indications:
  - Moderate renal failure.
  - Moderate aortic stenosis.

Adverse effects

- Cough (5–15%).
- Hypotension.
- Hyperkalaemia.
- Renal dysfunction.
- Angio-oedema.
- Bronchospasm.

✒ There is controversy regarding a possible interaction between aspirin and ACEIs, which might decrease the efficacy of the latter agents (Hall D. The aspirin-angiotensin-converting enzyme inhibitor tradeoff: to halve and halve not. *J Am Coll Cardiol* 2000; **35**: 1808–12).

Table 31.2 The titration steps for ACE inhibitors

Drug	Start dose (mg)	Uptitration steps (mg)	Target dose (mg)	Frequency
Captopril	6.25	12.5–25–50	50	tds
Enalapril	2.5	5–10–20	20	bd
Lisinopril	5	10–20–30–40	35–40	od
Ramipril	2.5	2.5	5	bd
Trandolapril	0.5	1–2–4	4	od

Clinical trial evidence base

Drugs that have been shown to reduce mortality in patients with chronic heart failure or LVSD include:

- Captopril.
- Enalapril.
- Lisinopril.
- Ramipril.
- Trandolapril.

There are a number of large RCTs of ACE inhibitors in patients with CHF. The main studies will be highlighted (Table 31.3).

Captopril

SAVE (survival and ventricular enlargement study)

Design: Double-blind RCT of captopril versus placebo in patients with LVSD 3–16 days post-MI

Subjects: $n = 2231$; Post-MI; LVEF < 40%; mean age = 59 years

Mean follow-up: 3.5 years

Results: 19% RRR in all-cause mortality (p = 0.019)

25% RRR in recurrent MI (p = 0.015)

32% RRR in death after recurrent MI

Reference: Pfeffer *et al.* Effect of captopril on morality and morbidity in patients with left ventricular dysfunction after myocardial infarction. Results of the survival and ventricular enlargement trial. The SAVE Investigators. *N Engl J Med* 1992; **327**: 669–77. Rutherford JD *et al.* Effects of captopril on ischemic events after myocardial infarction. Results of the Survival and Ventricular Enlargement trial. SAVE Investigators. *Circulation* 1994; **90**: 1731–8.

Table 31.3 Summary of ACE inhibitor RCTs in CHF/LVSD

Trial (Drug versus placebo)	Number of patients	NYHA class	Mean LVEF (%)	Mean follow-up (years)	Mortality reduction (%)	Withdrawal due to intolerance (% versus placebo)
SAVE Captopril	2231	Post-MI LVSD		3.5	19	—
CONSENSUS Enalapril	253	IV	—	0.5	40	14% versus 17%
SOLVD Enalapril	2569	90% II/III	27	3.4	16	—
ATLAS Lisinopril—Low versus high dose	3164	16% II 77% III 7% IV	23	3.8	—	17% versus 18%
AIRE Ramipril	2006	Post-MI HF	—	1.25	27	35% versus 32%
TRACE Trandolapril	1749	Post-MI LVSD	—	2.4	22	37% versus 36%

Enalapril

CONSENSUS (cooperative North Scandinavian enalapril survival study)
  Design: Double-blind RCT of enalapril versus placebo
  Subjects: n = 253; NYHA IV; mean age = 70.5 years; 70.5% ♂
  Mean follow-up: 0.5 year
  Results: 27% RRR in all-cause mortality (p = 0.003)
  Reference: Effects of enalapril on mortality in severe congestive heart
            failure. Results of the Cooperative North Scandinavian
            Enalapril Survival Study (CONSENSUS). The CONSENSUS
            Trial Study Group. N Engl J Med 1987; **316**: 1429–35.

SOLVD-Treatment
  Design: Double-blind RCT of enalapril versus placebo
  Subjects: n = 2569; LVEF ≤ 35%
  Mean follow-up: 3.4 years
  Results: 16% RRR in all-cause mortality (p = 0.0036)[1]
          26% RRR in death or hospitalization (p < 0.0001)[1]
          78% RRR in development of AF[2]
  Reference: Effect of enalapril on survival in patients with reduced left
            ventricular ejection fractions and congestive heart failure.
            The SOLVD Investigators. N Engl J Med 1991; **325**: 293–302
            Vermes et al. Enalapril decreases the incidence of atrial
            fibrillation in patients with left ventricular dysfunction:
            insight from the Studies Of Left ventricular Dysfunction
            (SOLVD) trials. Circulation 2003; **107**: 2926–31.

Lisinopril

ATLAS (assessment of treatment with lisinopril and survival)
  Design: Randomized comparison study of low- (2.5–5mg) and
          high- (32.5–35mg) dose lisinopril
  Subjects: n = 3164; NYHA II-IV; LVEF ≤ 30%; mean age = 64 years;
          80% ♂
  Mean follow-up: 3.8 years
  Results: 12% RRR in all-cause mortality or hospitalization (p = 0.002)
  No significant reduction in mortality (p = 0.13)
  Reference: Packer M et al. Comparative effects of low and high doses
            of the angiotensin-converting enzyme inhibitor, lisinopril,
            on morbidity and mortality in chronic heart failure. ATLAS
            Study Group. Circulation 1999; **100**: 2312–18.

Ramipril

AIRE (the acute infarction ramipril efficacy study)
  Design: Double-blind RCT of ramipril versus placebo in patients
          3–10 days post-MI with evidence of heart failure
  Subjects: n = 2006; LVEF ≤ 35%; mean age = 65 years; 74% ♂
  Mean follow-up: 1.25 years
  Results: 27% RRR in all-cause mortality (p = 0.002)
  Reference: Lancet 1993; **342**: 821–8.

Trandolapril

TRACE (trandolapril cardiac evaluation study)

Design: Double-blind RCT of trandolapril versus placebo in patients
3–7 days post-MI with evidence of LVSD

Subjects: n = 1749; LVEF ≤ 35%; mean age = 67.5 years; 71.5% ♂

Mean follow-up: approximately 3 years

Results: 22% RRR in all-cause mortality (p = 0.001)
24% RRR in sudden death (p = 0.03)
29% RRR in progression to severe HF (p = 0.003)

Reference: Kober L et al. A clinical trial of the angiotensin-converting-
enzyme inhibitor trandolapril in patients with left ventricular
dysfunction after myocardial infarction. Trandolapril Cardiac
Evaluation (TRACE) Study Group. N Engl J Med 1995; **333**:
1670–6.

β-adrenoreceptor antagonists

The adrenoreceptors

The concept of adrenoreceptors can be dated back to Langley in 1905. The theory of reducing myocardial oxygen demand in angina by antagonizing the β-adrenoreceptor was conceived by Sir James Black, and in 1958 dichloroisoprenaline was discovered, which is generally regarded as the first β-adrenoreceptor antagonist. Since then, many more such compounds have been created with differing affinities for the adrenoreceptors (Table 32.1), which have subsequently been classified as:

α_1-adrenoreceptors
• Post-synaptic.
• Stimulation causes peripheral vasoconstriction and venoconstriction.

α_2-adrenoreceptors
• Pre-synaptic.
• Stimulation causes pre-synaptic sympathetic inhibition.

β_1-adrenoreceptors
• Found mainly in the heart, intestine, and renin-secreting tissue of the kidney.
• Stimulation causes positive chronotropy and inotropy and increased a-v conduction.

β_2-adrenoreceptors
• Present predominantly in bronchial and vascular smooth muscle.
• Also found in GI tract, uterus, pancreas, and heart.
• Stimulation causes bronchial dilatation and peripheral vasodilatation.

The heart contains β-adrenoreceptors in the ratio 70% β_1:30% β_2.

Table 32.1 Actions of commonly used β-adrenoreceptor antagonists in CHF

Drug	α_1	β_1	β_2	Other properties
Bisoprolol	–	+++	–	–
Carvedilol	+	++	+	Antioxidant
Metoprolol	–	++	–	–
Nebivolol	–	++	–	Activate nitric oxide

The sympathetic nervous system in heart failure

Deleterious effects of the sympathetic nervous system in heart failure

- ↑ HR, contractility.
- Electrical instability.
- Apoptosis.
- Myocardial toxicity.
- LV dilatation and hypertrophy.
- Renin release.

Mechanism of action of β-adrenoreceptor antagonism in CHF

- Reduction in:
  - Renin release.
  - Angiotensin-II and aldosterone.
  - Myocardial oxygen demand.
  - Catecholamine-induced free fatty acid release from adipose tissue.
  - Myocardial oxidative stress.
- Improvement in cardiac function.
- Anti-arrhythmic effect.

Proven benefits of β-adrenoreceptor antagonism in CHF

- Reduction in all-cause mortality.
- Reduction in sudden cardiac death and pump failure.
- Improvement in left ventricular ejection fraction.
- Improvement in medium–long-term morbidity (with the possibility of short-term deterioration).
- Reduction in hospitalization.
- Reduction in the need for cardiac transplantation.
- May reduce cases of new-onset diabetes mellitus.

Pharmacokinetics

The major determinant of the pharmacokinetics of β-adrenoreceptor antagonists is their lipid solubility (Table 32.2).

Lipophilic β-adrenoreceptor antagonists (e.g. nebivolol) are generally:
- Well absorbed from the GI tract.
- Metabolized in the liver.
- Large volume of distribution (Vd), including across the blood-brain barrier (therefore can cause sleep disturbance).
- Highly protein bound.
- Short-acting.

Hydrophilic β-adrenoreceptor antagonists (e.g. atenolol) are generally:
- Less well absorbed from the GI tract.
- Excreted virtually unchanged by the kidney (therefore caution in renal impairment).
- Lower volume of distribution (in particular less likely to cross blood–brain barrier).
- Low protein bound.
- Longer-acting.

Clinical trial evidence base

The β-adrenoreceptor antagonists that have been sh_
outcome in patients with chronic heart failure include:
- Bisoprolol.
- Carvedilol.
- Metoprolol (succinate) XL.
- Nebivolol.

There are a number of large RCTs of β-adrenoreceptor blo_
patients with CHF. The main studies are highlighted (Table 32.4).

Bisoprolol

CIBIS (cardiac insufficiency bisoprolol study)

Design: Double-blind RCT of bisoprolol versus placebo
Subjects: n = 641; NYHA III/IV; LVEF < 40%; mean age = 60 years;
83% ♂
Follow-up: 1.9 years
Results: No significant difference in mortality (p = 0.22)
31% RRR in hospitalization (p < 0.01)
Improvement in NYHA functional class
Reference: A randomized trial of beta-blockade in heart failure. T_
Cardiac Insufficiency Bisoprolol Study (CIBIS). CIBIS Inv_
tigators and Committees. *Circulation* 1994; **90**: 1765–73.

CIBIS II (cardiac insufficiency bisoprolol study II)

Design: Double-blind RCT of bisoprolol versus placebo
Subjects: n = 2647; NYHA III/IV; LVEF ≤ 35%; mean age = 61 years;
88% ♂
Mean follow-up: 1.3 years
Results: 34% RRR of all-cause mortality (p < 0.0001)
44% RRR in sudden death (p = 0.0011)
20% RRR in hospitalization (p = 0.0006)
Reference: Simon *et al.* The cardiac insufficiency bisoprolol study
(CIBIS-II): a randomised trial. *Lancet* 1999; **353**: 9–13.

Carvedilol

US Carvedilol

Design: Double-blind RCT of carvedilol versus placebo (2:1)
Subjects: n = 366; NYHA II/III; LVEF ≤ 35%; mean age = 60 years;
85% ♂
Mean follow-up: 0.6 year
Results: 48% RRR in HF progression (p = 0.008)
77% RRR all-cause mortality (p = 0.048)
Reference: Colucci *et al.* Carvedilol inhibits clinical progression in
patients with mild symptoms of heart failure. US Carvedilo_
Heart Failure Study Group. *Circulation* 1996; **94**: 2800–6.

Table 32.2 The pharmacokinetics of β-adrenoreceptor antagonists

β-blocker	Bio-availability (%)	Plasma protein binding (%)	Lipid solubility	Half-life (hours)	Metabolism and elimination
Bisoprolol	90	30	Moderate	10–12	50% hepatic metabolism; renal excretion
Carvedilol	25	98	Moderate	6–10	Extensive hepatic metabolism; faecal excretion
Metoprolol	50–75	12	Moderate	3–7	Hepatic metabolism; faecal excretion
Nebivolol	12–100	98	High	10–50	Hepatic metabolism; faecal excretion
Atenolol*	50	10	Low	6–10	Renal excretion

▶* Atenolol does not have an evidence base in patients with chronic heart failure, but is displayed here for comparison and because many patients with CHF are already on this drug.

How to initiate (see also Chapter 5)

- Recommended in NYHA I–IV CHF.
- Patients should be euvolaemic.
- 'Start low, go slow'.
- Monitor heart rate, blood pressure, and for signs of fluid retention.
  - Aim for pulse >50/min and systolic BP >90mmHg.
- Double dose every 1–4 weeks if tolerated.
- Aim for target dose (see Table 32.3).

▶ A small dose is better than no dose at all!

Contra-indications to initiation

- Asthma.
- Significant bradycardia (<50/min).
- Mobitz type II or complete heart block.
- Cardiac decompensation.
- The following are not absolute contra-indications:
  - COPD without significant reversibility.
  - PVD.

Adverse effects

- Bradycardia/heart block.
- Hypotension.
- Cold extremities.
- Fluid retention (treat with diuretics).
- Fatigue.
- Masking of symptoms of hypoglycaemia.
- Initial worsening of symptoms including breathlessness (often improves).
- Sexual dysfunction.
- Sleep disturbance (particularly lipophilic drugs).

⚠ Abrupt discontinuation

Due to the upregulation of β-adrenoreceptors during treatment with β-adrenoreceptor antagonists, abrupt discontinuation can lead to:

- Arrhythmia.
- Exacerbation of angina.
- Worsening pump failure.
- Reflex hypertension.

Table 32.3 The titration steps for β-adrenoreceptor antagonists

g	Start dose (mg)	Uptitration steps (mg)	Target dose (mg)	Frequ
rvedilol	3.125	6.25–12.5–25–50*	25/50*	bd
soprolol	1.25	2.5–5–7.5–10	10	od
letoprolol[†] CR/XL	12.5[†]/25	25–50–100–200	200	od
Nebivolol	1.25	2.5–5–10	10	od

* Where patient is >85kg.
[†] Preparation not available in the UK.

Table 32.4 Summary of RCTs of β-adrenoreceptor antagonists in CHF

Trial (drug versus placebo)	Number of patients	NYHA class	Mean LVEF (%)	Mean follow-up (years)	Mortality reduction (%)	Increase in LVEF (%)	Withdrawal due to intolerance (% versus placebo)
CIBIS Bisoprolol	641	95% III 5% IV	25	1.9	–	–	23 versus 26
CIBIS-II Bisoprolol	2647	83% III 17% IV	28	1.3	34	–	15 versus 15
US Carvedilol	389	85% II 15% III	23	0.6	77	10	7.3 versus 10.4
Aus/NZ Carvedilol	415	30% I 54% II 16% III	28	1.6	–	5.3	17.6 versus 14.6
MOCHA Carvedilol	345	46% II 52% III 2% IV	23	0.5	73	8*	11 versus 13
Copernicus Carvedilol	2289	IV	19	0.9	39	–	14.8 versus 18.5

COMET Carvedilol versus metoprolol	3029	48% II 48% III 4% IV	26	4.8	17	–	32 versus 32
MERIT-HF Metoprolol	3991	41% II 55% III 4% IV	28	1.0	34	–	9.8 versus 11.7
SENIORS Nebivolol	2128	3% I 56% II 39% III 2% IV	36	1.8	–	–	26.7 versus 24.6

* In a dose-response manner with greatest improvement on 25mg bd.

Australia/New Zealand
  Design: Double-blind RCT of carvedilol versus placebo
  Subjects: n = 415; NYHA I–III; LVEF < 45%; mean age = 67 years;
      80% ♂
  Mean follow-up: 1.6 years
  Results: 26% RRR of all-cause mortality or hospitalization (p = 0.02)
      5.3% improvement in LVEF
  Reference: Randomised, placebo-controlled trial of carvedilol in
      patients with congestive heart failure due to ischaemic
      heart disease. Australia/New Zealand Heart Failure
      Research Collaborative Group. *Lancet* 1997; **349**: 375–80.

MOCHA
  Design: Double-blind dose-response evaluation of carvedilol versus
      placebo
  Subjects: n = 345; NYHA II–IV; LVEF < 35%; mean age = 60 years;
      76% ♂
  Mean follow-up: 0.5 year
  Results: Dose-dependent improvements in LVEF (p < 0.001)
      73% RRR all-cause mortality (p < 0.001).
  Reference: Bristow *et al.* Carvedilol produces dose-related
      improvements in left ventricular function and survival in
      subjects with chronic heart failure. MOCHA Investigators.
      Circulation 1996; **94**: 2807–16.

COPERNICUS (carvedilol prospective randomized cumulative survival study)
  Design: Double-blind RCT of carvedilol versus placebo
  Subjects: n = 2289; NYHA IV; LVEF < 25%; mean age = 63 years;
      80% ♂
  Mean follow-up: 10.4 months
  Results: 35% RRR of all-cause mortality (p = 0.0014)
      24% RRR of all-cause mortality/hospitalization (p < 0.001)
  Reference: Packer *et al.* Effect of carvedilol on survival in severe
      chronic heart failure. *N Engl J Med* 2001; **344**: 1651–8.

COMET (carvedilol or metoprolol European trial)
  Design: Double-blind RCT of carvedilol versus metoprolol tartrate🖙
  Subjects: n = 3029; NYHA II–IV; LVEF < 35%; mean age = 62 years;
      80% ♂
  Mean follow-up: 58 months
  Results: 17% RRR of all-cause mortality in carvedilol group (p = 0.0017)
  Reference: Poole-Wilson *et al.* Comparison of carvedilol and
      metoprolol on clinical outcomes in patients with chronic
      heart failure in the Carvedilol Or Metoprolol European
      Trial (COMET): randomised controlled trial. *Lancet* 2003;
      362: 7–13.

🖙Contentious issue regarding the formulation and doses of metoprolol
used.

Metoprolol
▶ Evidence base is only for metoprolol succinate not tartrate, which is the shorter-acting preparation available in the United Kingdom.

MERIT-HF (metoprolol CR/XL randomized interventional trial in heart failure)
    Design: Double-blind RCT of metoprolol succinate versus placebo
    Subjects: n = 3991; NYHA II–IV; LVEF ≤ 40%; mean age = 64 years; 78% ♂
    Mean follow-up: 12 months (terminated early)
    Results: 34% RRR of all-cause mortality (p = 0.00009)
            41% RRR in sudden death (p = 0.0002)
            19% RRR in all-cause mortality/hospitalization (p < 0.01)
    References: Effect of metoprolol CR/XL in chronic heart failure: Metoprolol CR/XL Randomised Intervention Trial in Congestive Heart Failure (MERIT-HF). *Lancet* 1999; **353**: 2001–7 and Hjalmarson A *et al.* Effects of controlled-release metoprolol on total mortality, hospitalizations, and well-being in patients with heart failure: the Metoprolol CR/XL Randomized Intervention Trial in congestive heart failure (MERIT-HF). MERIT-HF Study Group. *JAMA* 2000; **283**: 1295–302.

Nebivolol
SENIORS (study of the effects of nebivolol intervention on outcomes and re-hospitalization in seniors with heart failure)
    Design: Double-blind RCT of nebivolol versus placebo in patients over 70 years; LVEF ≤ 35% or admission with heart failure in previous 6 months
    Subjects: n = 2128; NYHA I–IV; mean age = 76 years; 63%♂
    Mean follow-up: 21 months
    Results: 14% RRR of all-cause mortality or cardiovascular hospital admission (p = 0.039)
            No significant difference in mortality (p = 0.21)
    Reference: Flather *et al.* Randomized trial to determine the effect of nebivolol on mortality and cardiovascular hospital admission in elderly patients with heart failure (SENIORS). *Eur Heart J* 2005; **26**: 215–25.

Aldosterone antagonists

Introduction

The final process in the renin–angiotensin–aldosterone system (RAAS) is the production of the mineralocorticoid aldosterone in the adrenal glands (Fig. 33.1). Aldosterone has an important role in the pathophysiology of heart failure. By acting on the distal convoluting tubule and collecting ducts in the kidney, aldosterone is a major regulator of extracellular fluid volume. It promotes the re-absorption of sodium, and is an important determinant of potassium and magnesium excretion. Aldosterone also causes sympathetic activation, parasympathetic inhibition, myocardial and vascular fibrosis, baroreceptor dysfunction, and impairment of arterial compliance.

It is well known that ACE inhibitors and ARBs only transiently suppress the production of aldosterone. Other mechanisms are involved in the mechanism of aldosterone release, including the response of the adrenal cortex to changes in K^+ concentration, as well as the action of adreno-corticotrophic hormone (ACTH). This has led to the successful trial of aldosterone antagonists in patients with NYHA class III/IV heart failure and in post-MI heart failure.

Proven benefits of aldosterone antagonism in CHF

- Reduction in mortality.
- Reduction in hospitalization for worsening CHF.
- Improvement in functional class.

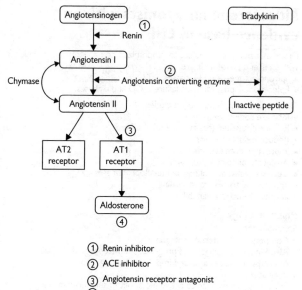

① Renin inhibitor
② ACE inhibitor
③ Angiotensin receptor antagonist
④ Aldosterone antagonist

Fig. 33.1 The sites of action of antagonists of the RAAS.

Aldosterone antagonists with an evidence base in CHF

Drugs that have been subject to randomized controlled trials in patients with CHF and post-MI HF are:
- Spironolactone—NYHA classes III/IV.
- Eplerenone—post MI heart failure/LVSD and diabetes.

The properties of these drugs include:
- Increase sodium excretion.
- Reduce potassium loss at distal renal tubule.
- Reduce oxidative stress.
- Improve endothelial function.
- Attenuate platelet aggregation.
- Decrease activation of matrix metalloproteinases.
- Improve ventricular re-modelling.
- Improve heart-rate variability.

Pharmacology

Spironolactone
- Competitive aldosterone antagonist.
- Also binds to androgen and progesterone receptors, therefore can cause gynaecomastia and impotence among men.
- Well absorbed orally.
- Principally metabolized to active metabolites: sulphur-containing metabolites (80%) and canrenone (20%).
- Although the plasma half-life of spironolactone itself is short (1.3 hours), the half-lives of the active metabolites are longer (2.8–11.2 hours).
- Elimination of metabolites occurs primarily in the urine and secondarily through biliary excretion in the faeces.
- The renal action of a single dose of spironolactone reaches its peak after 7 hours, and activity persists for at least 24 hours.

Eplerenone
- Competitive selective aldosterone antagonist (greater selectivity for the mineralocorticoid receptor than spironolactone).
- Metabolism is primarily mediated via cytochrome P450 (CYP3A4).
- No active metabolites of eplerenone have been identified in human plasma.
- Less than 5% of an eplerenone dose is recovered as unchanged drug in urine and faeces. Following a single oral dose of radiolabelled drug, approximately 32% of the dose was excreted in faeces and approximately 67% was excreted in urine.
- The elimination half-life of eplerenone is approximately 3–5 hours.

Table 33.1 Pharmacokinetics of the aldosterone antagonists

Aldosterone antagonist	Bioavailability (%)	Plasma protein binding (%)	Half-life (hours)	Metabolism
Spironolactone	90	90	1.3	Extensively to active drug
Eplerenone	69	50	3–5	P450 (CYP3A4)

How to initiate (see also Chapter 5) (Table 33.2)

- Do not commence if the baseline creatinine is >220µmol/L.
- Monitor within 1 week after starting for renal dysfunction and hyperkalaemia.
- Use with caution in the elderly.
- Stop aldosterone antagonist temporarily during episodes of diarrhoea and/or vomiting.

Contra-indications to initiation

- Significant renal impairment.
- Hyperkalaemia.

Side-effects

- Hyponatraemia.
- Hyperkalaemia.
- Renal dysfunction.
- Gynaecomastia—spironolactone[*].
- Impotence—spironolactone[*].

Clinical trial evidence base (Table 33.3)

Spironolactone

RALES (Randomized aldactone evaluation study)
   Design: Double-blind RCT of spironolactone versus placebo
   Subjects: n = 1663; NYHA III/IV; LVEF ≤ 35%; mean age = 65 years; 73% ♂
   Follow-up: 2 years (discontinued early)
   Results: 30% RRR in mortality; 35% RRR in hospitalization for worsening CHF and improvement in functional class
   Reference: Pitt B et al. The effect of spironolactone on morbidity and mortality in patients with severe heart failure. Randomized Aldactone Evaluation Study Investigators. N Engl J Med 1999; **341**: 709–17.

Eplerenone

EPHESUS (Eplerenone post–acute myocardial infarction heart failure efficacy and survival study)
   Design: Double-blind RCT of eplerenone versus placebo
   Subjects: n = 6632; NYHA III/IV; LVEF < 40%; mean age = 64 years; 71% ♂
   Follow-up: 1.3 years
   Results: 15% RRR in mortality; 21% RRR of sudden death
   Reference: Pitt B et al. Eplerenone, a selective aldosterone blocker, in patients with left ventricular dysfunction after myocardial infarction. N Engl J Med 2003; **348**: 1309–21.

---

[*] Eplerenone can be substituted, but this is an unlicensed indication.

Table 33.2 Titration steps for the aldosterone antagonists

Drug	Start dose (mg)	Target dose (mg)	Frequency
Spironolactone	25	50	od
Eplerenone	25	50	od

Table 33.3 Summary of RCTs of aldosterone antagonists in CHF

Trial (drug versus placebo)	Number of patients	NYHA class (%)	Mean LVEF (%)	Mean follow-up (years)	Mortality reduction (%)	Withdrawal due to intolerance (% versus placebo)
RALES Spironolactone	1663	0.5 II 70.5 III 29 IV	25	1.9	30	8 versus 5
EPHESUS Eplerenone	6632	–	33	1.3	15	4 versus 3

Chapter 34

Angiotensin receptor antagonists

Introduction

The renin–angiotensin–aldosterone system (RAAS) is activated in patients with heart failure and, as mentioned in 📖 Chapter 2, contributes to many of the detrimental effects seen in these patients. The RAAS is not completely blocked by ACE inhibition, since angiotensin II is also produced through the mechanisms distinct from ACE pathways. The development of antagonists to the angiotensin II type-1 (AT_1)-receptor (ARBs) provides a pharmacologically different mechanism of inhibiting the RAAS (Fig. 34.1).

In theory, inhibition of the RAAS by blockade of the AT_1-receptor can result in a more complete inhibition of the adverse cardiovascular effects of angiotensin II, while the other potentially desirable actions modulated by different angiotensin-II receptors are potentially left unopposed. However, not all the effects of unopposed stimulation of the AT_2-receptor may be beneficial. Unlike ACE-inhibitors, ARBs do not inhibit bradykinin breakdown and thus are much less likely to cause side-effects associated with ACE inhibitors, such as cough, bronchospasm, and angio-oedema.

The effects of angiotensin II on the principle receptors are:

AT_1 receptor
- Vasoconstriction.
- Sodium and water retention.
- Aldosterone synthesis and secretion.
- Increased vasopressin secretion.
- Cardiac hypertrophy.

AT_2 receptor
- Inhibition of cell growth.
- Vasodilation.
- Apoptosis.
- Modulation of extracellular matrix.
- Cellular differentiation.

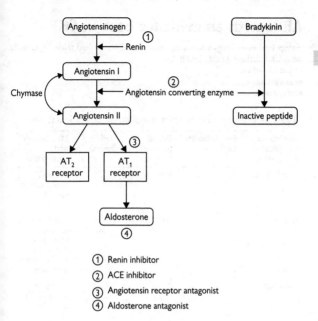

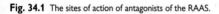

① Renin inhibitor
② ACE inhibitor
③ Angiotensin receptor antagonist
④ Aldosterone antagonist

Fig. 34.1 The sites of action of antagonists of the RAAS.

ARBs with an evidence base in CHF

Drugs that have been subject to randomized controlled trials in patients with CHF include (Table 34.1):
- Candesartan.
- Losartan.
- Valsartan.

Table 34.1 The pharmacokinetics of angiotensin receptor antagonists

Angiotensin receptor antagonists	Bioavailability (%)	Plasma protein binding (%)	Half-life (hours)	Metabolism and elimination
Candesartan	34	>99	9	Largely unchanged via urine and faeces
Losartan	33	>99	2 (6–9)[†]	14% converted to active metabolite; 35% urinary and 58% faecal excretion
Valsartan	23	94–97	1–9	Unchanged in faeces (83%) and urine (13%)
Irbesartan*	60–80	96	11–15	Hepatic metabolism via P450; 80% excreted unchanged in faeces

* Irbesartan does not have an evidence base in patients with CHF, but is displayed here for comparison.
[†] Active metabolite.

How to initiate (see also Chapter 5)

- Indicated in all CHF patients who are ACE-intolerant (unless contra-indication exists).
- The addition of candesartan to ACE inhibitor and β-adrenoreceptor antagonist in patients with NYHA II-III CHF should be considered
- Start at a low dose and uptitrate (Table 34.2).

Contra-indications to initiation

- Bilateral renal artery stenosis.
- Severe renal failure without renal replacement therapy.
- Pregnancy.

Side-effects

- Hypotension.
- Renal dysfunction.
- Hyperkalaemia.
- Hyponatraemia.

Table 34.2 The titration steps for angiotensin receptor antagonists

Drug	Start dose (mg)	Uptitration steps (mg)	Target dose (mg)	Frequency
Candesartan	4	8–16	32	od
Losartan*	25	50	100	od
Valsartan	40	80	160	bd
Irbesartan†	75	150	300	od

* Target dose in ELITE and ELITE II was 50mg od.
† Irbesartan does not have an evidence base in HF, but is being shown here for comparison.

Clinical trial evidence base

There are a number of large RCTs of angiotensin receptor antagonists in patients with CHF. The main studies will be highlighted (Table 34.3).

Candesartan

CHARM-Overall (candesartan in heart failure: assessment of reduction in mortality and morbidity)

Design: Double-blind RCT of candesartan versus placebo

Subjects: Three populations:

> LVEF < 40% intolerant to ACE inhibitors
> LVEF < 40% and already on ACE inhibitors
> LVEF > 40%
> In total: n = 7599; NYHA II–IV; mean age = 66 years; 68% ♂

Median follow-up: 3.1 years

Target dose = 32mg (Mean dose 24mg)

Results: 9% RRR in mortality (p = 0.055)

> 12% RRR in CV deaths (p = 0.012)
> 21% RRR in hospitalization for CHF (p < 0.0001)

Reference: Pfeffer MA et al. Effects of candesartan on mortality and morbidity in patients with chronic heart failure: the CHARM-Overall programme. Lancet 2003; **362**: 759–66.

CHARM-Alternative

Design: Double-blind RCT of candesartan versus placebo

Subjects: LVEF < 40% intolerant to ACE inhibitors; n = 2028; NYHA II–IV; mean age = 66 years; 68% ♂

Median follow-up: 2.8 years

Results: 23% RRR in CV death or CHF hospitalization (p = 0.0004)

> 32% RRR in hospitalization for CHF (p < 0.0001)

Reference: Granger CB et al. Effects of candesartan in patients with chronic heart failure and reduced left-ventricular systolic function intolerant to angiotensin-converting enzyme inhibitors: the CHARM-Alternative trial. Lancet 2003; **362**: 772–76.

CHARM-Added

Design: Double-blind RCT of candesartan versus placebo

Subjects: LVEF < 40%; on ACE inhibitor; n = 2548; NYHA II–IV; mean age = 64 years; 79% ♂

Median follow-up: 3.4 years

Results: 15% RRR in CV death or CHF hospitalization (p = 0.011)

> 17% RRR in hospitalization for CHF (p < 0.014)

Reference: McMurray JJ et al. Effects of candesartan in patients with chronic heart failure and reduced left-ventricular systolic function taking angiotensin-converting-enzyme inhibitors: the CHARM-Added trial. Lancet 2003; **362**: 767–71.

CHARM-Preserved
  Design: Double-blind RCT of candesartan versus placebo
  Subjects: LVEF > 40% in NYHA II–IV; n = 3023; mean age = 67 years;
      60% ♂
  Median follow-up: 3 years
  Results: Non-significant effect on CV death or CHF hospitalization on
      unadjusted hazard ratio
      No effect on CV death
  Reference: Yusuf, S et al. Effects of candesartan in patients with chronic
      heart failure and preserved left-ventricular ejection fraction:
      the CHARM-Preserved Trial. Lancet 2003; **362**: 777–81.

Table 34.3 Summary of RCTs of angiotensin receptor antagonists in CHF

Trial (Drug versus placebo)	Number of patients	NYHA class (%)	Mean LVEF (%)	Mean follow-up (years)	Mortality reduction (%)	Increase in LVEF (%)	Withdrawal due to intolerance (% versus placebo)
CHARM-Overall Candesartan	7599	45 II 52 III 3 IV	39	3.1	9*	–	23 versus 19
CHARM-Alternative Candesartan	2028	47 II 49 III 4 IV	30	2.8	17†	–	24 versus 22*
CHARM-Added Candesartan	2548	24 II 73 III 3 IV	28	3.4	–	–	25 versus 18
CHARM-Preserved Candesartan	3023	61 II 37 III 2 IV	54	3.0	–	–	22 versus 18
ELITE Losartan versus captopril	722	65 II 34 III 2 IV	31	0.9	–	–	18.5 versus 30
ELITE II Losartan versus captopril	3152	52 II 43 III 5 IV	31	1.5	–	–	10 versus 15
Val-HeFT Valsartan	5010	62 II 36 III 2 IV	27	1.9	–	4.5 versus 3.2	9.9 versus 7.7

* Not significant.
† Adjusted figures.

Losartan

ELITE (evaluation of losartan in the elderly study)
Design: Double-blind RCT of losartan versus captopril
Subjects: $n = 722$; LVEF $\leq 40\%$; NYHA II–IV; age ≥ 65 years; mean age
= 73.5 years; 67% ♂
Follow-up: 48 weeks
Target doses: 50mg losartan od; 50mg captopril tds
Mean daily dose: 42.6mg losartan; 122.7mg captopril
Results: Fewer drug discontinuations with losartan ($p = 0.002$)
No significant difference in death or hospitalization ($p = 0.075$)
No difference in renal dysfunction
Reference: Pitt B et al. Randomised trial of losartan versus captopril in
patients over 65 with heart failure (Evaluation of Losartan in
the Elderly Study, ELITE). Lancet 1997; **349**: 747–52.

ELITE II (evaluation of losartan in the elderly study)
Design: Double-blind RCT of losartan versus captopril
Subjects: $n = 3152$; LVEF $\leq 40\%$; NYHA II–IV; age ≥ 60 years; mean age
= 71 years; 70% ♂
Median follow-up: 1.5 years
Target doses: 50mg losartan od; 50mg captopril tds
Results: No difference in all-cause mortality
No difference in hospitalization
Fewer drug discontinuations with losartan ($p < 0.001$)
Reference: Pitt B et al. Effect of losartan compared with captopril on
mortality in patients with symptomatic heart failure:
randomised trial—the Losartan Heart Failure Survival Study
ELITE II. Lancet 2000; **355**: 1582–87.

Valsartan

Val-HeFT (valsartan-heart failure trial)
Design: Double-blind RCT of valsartan versus placebo
Subjects: $n = 5010$; LVEF $< 40\%$; NYHA II–IV; mean age = 63 years;
80% ♂
Target dose: 160mg bd; mean daily dose = 254mg
Background therapy: 93% ACE-i; 35% β-blocker; 5% spironolactone
Mean follow-up: 23 months
Results: No significant difference in mortality
13% RRR in combined endpoint (death, HF hospitalization,
IV therapy, cardiac arrest with resuscitation) ($p = 0.009$)
Adverse effect on mortality in patients receiving ACE-I and
β-blocker ($p = 0.009$)
Reference: Cohn, JN et al. A randomized trial of the angiotensin-
receptor blocker valsartan in chronic heart failure. N Engl J
Med 2001; **345**: 1667–75.

Diuretics

Introduction

Na^+ and Cl^- are the major determinants of extracellular fluid volume. Therefore, the role of diuretics is to increase the net loss of sodium and water by interfering with sodium, chloride, and water transport in the renal tubular cell membrane. As a large proportion of sodium and water that passes through the nephron is re-absorbed, even a small reduction in re-absorption can result in a marked increase in excretion.

Diuretics are commonly classified into the following groups (Fig. 35.1 and Table 35.1):
- Loop (e.g. furosemide, bumetanide).
- Thiazide (e.g. bendroflumethiazide).
- Aldosterone antagonists (e.g. spironolactone).
- Potassium-sparing (e.g. amiloride).
- Osmotic diuretics (e.g. mannitol).
- Carbonic anhydrase inhibitors (e.g. acetazolamide).

The latter group, the carbonic anhydrase inhibitors, have limited usefulness as diuretics. In contrast, loop diuretics form the cornerstone of therapy for patients with CHF and evidence of fluid retention. CHF patients may also require the addition of a thiazide to augment diuresis, and potentially overcome diuretic resistance that can often be seen with higher doses of loop diuretic.

▶ It is important to ensure that those patients with CHF who require diuretic therapy are commenced on an appropriate salt and fluid restriction (usually 1.5 L/day), and counselled on fluid balance and daily weights.

Diuretic resistance

Oedematous patients may exhibit apparent resistance to oral diuretics due to reduced intestinal drug absorption. Patients with renal insufficiency often exhibit 'diuretic resistance', that is, a markedly reduced diuretic response. At a GFR <30mL/minute, little of the filtered Na^+ and water reach the distal segments of the nephron. In addition, these patients are often more or less refractory to diuretics for several reasons:
- Renal hypoperfusion.
- Increased intraluminal protein binding of the diuretic.
- Reduced tubular secretion (renal failure, NSAIDs).
- Intravascular volume depletion.
- Neurohormonal activation.
- Hypertrophy of distal nephron.
- Tubuloglomerular feedback (mediated by adenosine α_1-receptor).
- Impaired gut absorption of an oral diuretic.
- Non-compliance with drugs or diet (high sodium intake).

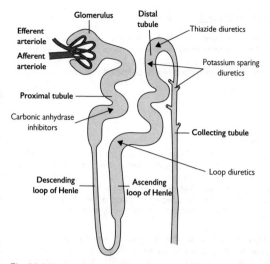

Fig. 35.1 The site of action of diuretics on the nephron.

Table 35.1 The pharmacokinetics of diuretics

Diuretic	Class	Bioavail-ability (%)	Onset of action, minutes (oral/iv)	t½ (hours)	Elimination (%)
Furosemide	Loop	52	40/5 Peak = 90	1½	60 R 40 M
Bumetanide	Loop	85	40/5 Peak = 90	1	65 R 35 M
Torasemide	Loop	85	40/10 Peak = 90	3	30 R 70 M
Bendro-flumethiazide	Thiazide	99	120/–	3	30 R 70 M
Metolazone	Thiazide	65	60/–	4–5	80 R 10 B 10 M
Spirono-lactone	Aldosterone antagonist	65	120/–	1.3	100 M
Amiloride	K⁺ sparing	50	120/–	6–9	100 R
Triamterene	K⁺ sparing	30–70	120/–	2	50 M 50 R

Abbreviations: R = Renal excretion of intact drug; B = excretion of intact drug into bile; M = Metabolized.

Loop diuretics

Loop diuretics are inhibitors of Na^+–K^+–$2Cl^-$ carrier in the luminal membrane of the cells of the thick ascending loop of Henle. They are the most powerful of all diuretics (often referred to as 'high ceiling diuretics'), capable of excreting approximately 20% of filtered sodium.

Examples of loop diuretics include:
- Furosemide.
- Bumetanide.
- Torasemide.

Administration

Table 35.2 has recommended starting doses of the principle loop diuretics. These can be titrated—both up and down—as required. High doses are sometimes necessary in patients with coexisting chronic renal failure. However, the lowest effective dose should be used at all times, in conjunction with a fluid restriction. Indeed, a retrospective study by Neuberg *et al.* suggests that high diuretic doses are an independent risk factor for mortality.

Once patients are on furosemide 80mg bd (or equivalent), the addition of a thiazide diuretic (e.g. bendroflumethiazide 2.5mg) is often preferable to escalating doses of loop diuretic, with careful monitoring of electrolytes and renal function.

Undesirable effects
- Hypokalaemia, hypocalcaemia, hypomagnesaemia, hyponatraemia.
- Hypotension.
- Hyperuricaemia.
- Metabolic alkalosis.
- Ototoxicity.

Table 35.2 The titration steps of loop diuretics

Loop diuretic	Equivalent doses (mg)	Starting dose	Maximum daily dose
Furosemide	40	40mg od	Titrated to response
Bumetanide	1	1mg od	Titrated to response
Torasemide	10	5mg od	Normal max 40mg (up to 200mg)

Reference

Neuberg GW *et al.* Diuretic resistance predicts mortality in patients with advanced heart failure. *Am Heart J* 2002; **144**: 31–8.

Thiazide diuretics

Thiazides exert their diuretic effect by inhibiting the active re-absorption of sodium and accompanying chloride in the early distal convoluted tubules, resulting in up to 10% of sodium in the filtrate being excreted. They, therefore, elicit a weaker diuretic response compared with the loop diuretics.

Examples of thiazide diuretics include:
• Bendroflumethiazide.
• Hydrochlorothiazide.
• Metolazone (see below).

Metolazone is a thiazide-like diuretic that primarily exerts its effects on the distal tubule. However, it also appears to have a significant proximal diuretic effect, which would increase the fraction of the filtered Na^+ that reaches the loop of Henle. This is potentially desirable in patients with a markedly reduced GFR, as metolazone also prevents any compensatory increase in distal Na^+ re-absorption.

Administration

Thiazide diuretics are generally not administered to heart failure patients, except those who are already established on loop diuretics, and require escalation of therapy due to fluid retention. This combination can result in a profound diuresis, and the patient should therefore be supervised closely, with the monitoring of renal function, electrolytes, and fluid status.

A thiazide, when added to a loop diuretic, should be tailored to each patient. Some only require, for example, bendroflumethiazide 2.5mg once weekly on top of their normal daily furosemide regimen of 80mg bd. Others may require daily thiazide administration (Table 35.3).

Undesirable effects
• Hypotension.
• Hypokalaemia, hypomagnesaemia, hyponatraemia.
• Hypercalcaemia.
• Hyperglycaemia.
• Pancreatitis.
• Metabolic alkalosis.

▶ Thiazide and loop diuretic combination therapy can cause a marked hyponatraemia or deterioration in renal function, and patients should be monitored closely.

Table 35.3 The titration steps of thiazide diuretics

Thiazide diuretic	Relative potency	Starting dose	Maximum daily dose
Bendroflumethiazide	10	2.5mg thrice weekly	10mg od mane
Hydrochlorothiazide	1	12.5mg od	50mg
Metolazone	10	2.5mg thrice weekly	20mg od mane

Potassium-sparing diuretics

Potassium-sparing diuretics are of limited diuretic efficacy, causing excretion of about 5% of the sodium in the filtrate. They include amiloride, triamterene, and spironolactone. Their principle sites of action are the distal convoluted tubule and the collecting tubules, inhibiting both sodium re-absorption and potassium excretion.

Amiloride and triamterene act by blocking the Na^+ channels in the luminal membrane of the principal cells of the cortical collecting ducts. This reduces the Na^+ entry through the luminal membrane, and hence the net re-absorption of NaCl. Spironolactone is a competitive aldosterone antagonist, which is discussed in more detail in 📖 Chapter 33.

Administration

Amiloride and triamterene are occasionally used for their *potassium-sparing* properties, in addition to, for example, a loop diuretic (Table 35.4). However, hypokalaemia in heart failure patients can usually be managed with the use of ACE inhibitors and/or angiotensin receptor antagonists, and aldosterone antagonists.

Undesirable effects

- Hyperkalaemia.
- Hyponatramia.
- Postural hypotension.
- GI disturbance.
- Dry mouth.
- Photosensitivity.

Table 35.4 Titration steps of potassium sparing diuretics

K$^+$ sparing diuretic	Starting dose	Maximum daily dose
Amiloride	5mg od	20mg od
Triamterene	150mg alt days	250mg od
Spironolactone	25mg od	400mg od

Inotropes and vasopressors

Principles of inotropes

Inotropes are often used to offer haemodynamic support to patients with decompensated heart failure. Although several drugs with inotropic activity are available, it has become increasingly evident that these drugs are associated with important negative effects. The positive inotropic actions of many of these agents are based on increased intracellular calcium concentrations, which may enhance myocardial energy consumption and arrhythmias.

Inotropic agents are classified according to their mode of action:
- β-adrenergic agonists—induce an increase in intracellular cAMP activity by the stimulation of cellular receptors.
- Dopexamine.
- Cardiac glycosides.
- Phosphodiesterase inhibitors.
- Calcium sensitizers.

Dobutamine

Dobutamine is a synthetic catecholamine with β_1-, β_2-, and α_1-adrenergic activity.

Properties
- Inotropic.
- Chronotropic.
- Vasodilator at higher doses.

Undesirable effects
- Increases myocardial oxygen demand.
- Pro-arrhythmic secondary to abnormal calcium loading.
- Leads to hypotension at higher doses.
- Tachyphylaxis—prolonged infusion over 96 hours has been associated with a decrease in the haemodynamic effect by as much as 50%.

Pharmacology
- Onset of action 1–2 minutes; peak effect within 10 minutes.
- Plasma half-life is 2 minutes.
- Metabolites are excreted via kidneys.

Common interactions
There is a risk of severe hypertension with
- β-adrenoreceptor antagonists (unopposed $\alpha1$-adrenergic activity).
- Monoamine oxidase inhibitors (MAOIs).

Administration
- Ideally should be given centrally due to possible phlebitis.
- Administered in doses from 2.5–25µg/kg/minute (see Tables 36.1 and 36.2).

Beneficial short-term action encouraged investigators to use the drug in patients with CHF on an out-patient basis. Intermittent therapy was found to increase the quality of life and haemodynamics. However, a clinical trial had to be stopped prematurely because of an increase in mortality in the dobutamine-treated group.

Table 36.1 Infusion chart for dobutamine

| | Dobutamine (2mg/mL) infusion rate (mL/hour) | | | | | | | |
| | Patient body weight (kg) | | | | | | | |
Dose (µg/kg/minute)	40	50	60	70	80	90	100	110
2.5	3	4	4.5	5	6	7	7.5	8
5	6	7.5	9	10.5	12	13.5	15	16.5
7.5	9	11	13.5	16	18	20	22.5	25
10	12	15	18	21	24	27	30	33
15	18	22.5	27	31.5	36	40.5	45	49.5
20	24	30	36	42	48	54	60	66
25	30	37.5	45	52.5	60	67.5	75	82.5

500mg of dobutamine made up to 250mL with either 5% dextrose or 0.9% saline.

Table 36.2 Infusion chart for dobutamine

| | Dobutamine (1mg/mL) infusion rate (mL/hour) | | | | | | | |
| | Patient body weight (kg) | | | | | | | |
Dose (µg/kg/minute)	40	50	60	70	80	90	100	110
2.5	6	7.5	9	10.5	12	13.5	15	16.5
5	12	15	18	21	24	27	30	33
7.5	18	22.5	27	31.5	36	40.5	45	49.5
10	24	30	36	42	48	54	60	66
15	36	45	54	63	72	81	90	99
20	48	60	72	84	96	108	120	132
25	60	75	90	105	120	135	140	155

250mg of dobutamine made up to 250mL with either 5% dextrose or 0.9% saline.

Dopamine

Dopamine is an endogenous precursor of norepinephrine, with predominantly β_1-receptor activity. However, at low doses, it acts on dopamine receptors (DA_1) causing dilation of smooth muscles in renal arteries, which can augment diuresis in combination with diuretics. At higher doses, it has inotropic effects through β_1 receptors, and vasoconstrictor effects via α_1 and 5HT receptors.

Properties (see above)
- May augment diuresis.
- Inotropic.
- Minor effects on heart rate or blood pressure except at higher doses.

Undesirable effects
- Extravasation may cause local necrosis.
- Pro-arrhythmic secondary to abnormal calcium loading.

Pharmacology
- Steady state reached within 5–10 minutes.
- Plasma half-life of 9 minutes.
- Widely distributed throughout the body.
- Does not cross the blood/brain barrier.
- Metabolized by monoamine oxidase (MAO) and catechol-O-methyl transerase (COMT), in the liver, kidney, and plasma.

Common interactions

Potentiated by:
- Monoamine oxidase inhibitors (MAOIs). In patients who have received MAOIs within the previous 2–3 weeks, the initial dopamine dose should be no greater than 10% of the usual dose.
- Tricyclic antidepressants.

Antagonized by:
- β-adrenoreceptor antagonists.

Hypotension and bradycardia have been observed in patients receiving phenytoin.

Administration
- Ideally through a central vein to avoid extravasation (Tables 36.3 and 36.4).
- To augment diuresis in patients with decompensated HF, use at low dose with IV diuretics (diuretic-dose dopamine).
- Do not discontinue abruptly—decrease dose gradually.

Table 36.3 The dose-dependent effects of dopamine

Dose	0.5–3.0 µg/kg/minute	3.0–5.0 µg/kg/minute	>5.0 µg/kg/minute
Predominant action	DA_1	β_1	5HT and α_1
Cardiovascular	↑ Cardiac output	↑ Myocardial contractility	↑ Heart rate vasoconstriction
Renal	↓ Proximal tubular Na re-absorption ↑ Renal blood flow	↑ Renal blood flow	Variable effect on renal blood flow
Gastrointestinal	↑ Splanchnic blood flow	↑ Splanchnic blood flow	Variable effect on splanchnic blood flow

Table 36.4 Infusion chart for dopamine

	Dopamine (1.6mg/mL) infusion rate (mL/hour)							
	Patient body weight (kg)							
Dose (µg/kg/minute)	40	50	60	70	80	90	100	110
2.5	4	5	6	7	8	8	9	10
5	8	9	11	13	15	17	19	20
7.5	12	14	17	20	23	25	28	30
10	15	19	23	26	30	34	38	39
15	23	28	34	39	45	51	56	59
20	30	38	45	53	60	68	75	79

400mg dopamine made up to 250mL with 5% dextrose or 0.9% saline.

Epinephrine (adrenaline)

Epinephrine is a direct-acting sympathomimetic agent, exerting its effect on β_1, β_2, and α_1 adrenoreceptors. Generally, it does not have a role in the management of acute heart failure.

Properties
- Inotropic.
- Chronotropic.
- Vasoconstriction.
- Bronchodilator.

Undesirable effects
- Increases myocardial oxygen demand.
- Pro-arrhythmic secondary to abnormal calcium loading.
- Hypertension.
- Hyperglycaemia.
- Hypokalaemia.
- Increased renin secretion.
- Increased after-load.
- Reduction in renal blood flow with higher doses.

Pharmacology
- Rapid onset of action.
- Plasma half-life is 5–10 minutes.
- 50% protein bound.
- Rapidly metabolized in the liver and tissues and excreted in the urine.

Administration
- Use with extreme caution.
- Indicated in cardiac arrest or in severe cardiogenic shock with haemodynamic monitoring (Table 36.5).

Table 36.5 Infusion chart for epinephrine

| Dose (μg/kg/minute) | Epinephrine (16μg/mL) infusion rate (mL/hour) | | | | | | | |
| | Patient body weight (kg) | | | | | | | |
	40	50	60	70	80	90	100	110
0.03	4.5	6	7	8	9	10	11	12
0.05	7.5	9	11	13	15	17	19	21
0.1	15	19	23	26	30	34	38	41
0.2	30	38	45	52	60	68	75	83
0.3	45	57	68	78	90	102	114	124
0.4	60	75	90	104	120	135	150	165
0.5	75	94	112	130	150	169	188	206

4mg epinephrine made up to 250mL with 5% dextrose. At larger doses and therefore volumes, the concentration of the infusion can be increased (double strength, triple strength, etc.), thereby reducing the necessary infusion rate and volume load to patient.

Norepinephrine (noradrenaline)

Norepinephrine is an endogenous agonist at α_1 and α_2 adrenoreceptors. It has a modest effect on β_1 adrenoreceptors. Generally, it does not have a role in the management of acute heart failure, as SVR is usually high in these patients.

Properties
- Vasoconstriction.

Undesirable effects
- Reduced renal blood flow.
- Splanchnic and distal limb ischaemia.
- Increased pulmonary vascular resistance.
- Uterine contraction.
- Metabolic acidosis.
- Arrhythmia secondary to abnormal calcium loading.

Pharmacology
- Inactive orally.
- Extensively metabolized.
- Only small amounts are excreted unchanged in the urine.

Administration
- Use with extreme caution
- Administer centrally with haemodynamic monitoring
- Dilute in 5% dextrose
- Initial infusion rates are between 2 and 12µg/minute (Table 36.6)
- Indicated in septic shock

Table 36.6 Infusion chart for norepinephrine

Dose (µg/kg/minute)	Norepinephrine infusion rate (mL/hour)							
	Patient body weight (kg)							
	40	**50**	**60**	**70**	**80**	**90**	**100**	**110**
0.03	4.5	6	7	8	9	10	11	12
0.05	7.5	9	11	13	15	17	19	21
0.1	15	19	23	26	30	34	38	41
0.2	30	38	45	52	60	68	75	83
0.3	45	57	68	78	90	102	114	124
0.4	60	75	90	104	120	135	150	165
0.5	75	94	112	130	150	169	188	206
1.0	150	186	224	260	300	338	375	412

4mg norepinephrine made up to 250mL with 5% dextrose (16µg/mL). At larger doses and therefore volumes, the concentration of the infusion can be increased (double strength, triple strength, etc.), thereby reducing the necessary infusion rate and volume load to patient.

Dopexamine

Dopexamine is a synthetic analogue of dopamine. It stimulates adrenergic β_2-receptors and peripheral dopamine receptors, and inhibits the neuronal re-uptake of noradrenaline.

Properties
- Increase in cardiac output mediated by after-load reduction (β_2, DA1).
- Mildly inotropic (β_2, uptake-1 inhibition).
- Increase in blood flow to vascular beds (DA1) such as the renal and mesenteric beds.
- Does not cause vasoconstriction.

Undesirable effects
- Tachycardia/tachyarrhythmia.
- Hypertension.

Pharmacology
- Rapid onset of action.
- Plasma half-life of around 11 minutes in patients with cardiac failure.
- Subsequent elimination of the metabolites is by urinary and biliary excretion.

Common interactions
- Enhances effects of epinephrine and norepinephrine.
- Risk of hypertensive crisis with MAOIs.

Administration
- By intravenous infusion into central or large peripheral vein.
- Dose: 0.5–6µg/kg/minute.

Cardiac glycosides

Cardiac glycosides increase the force of myocardial contraction and reduce conductivity within the atrioventricular (AV) node. The most commonly used cardiac glycoside is digoxin, although its role in heart failure is not clear. The current recommendations (**not** based on evidence) are to introduce this drug in patients who remain symptomatic, despite maximal, medical therapy or to provide rate control for patients with atrial fibrillation (AF).

Indications
- Symptomatic improvement in advanced chronic heart failure (in patients already established on maximally tolerated disease-modifying therapy—📖 see Chapter 6), aiming for serum digoxin concentrations of 0.65–1.0nmol/L (0.5–0.8ng/mL).
- The control of ventricular rate in persistent atrial fibrillation (as an adjunct to beta-blockade).

Undesirable effects
- Narrow therapeutic window.
- Multiple side-effects.
- Pro-arrhythmic.
- Dose adjustment made in renal impairment.

Toxicity
- Discontinue digoxin.
- Digibind (digoxin-specific antibody fragments) can be given for more haemodynamically significant digoxin toxicity.

Important interactions
- Increased cardiac toxicity with digoxin and hypokalaemia.
- The plasma concentration of digoxin is increased with:
  - Amiodarone—half dose of digoxin.
  - Propafenone and quinidine.
  - Diltiazem, verapamil, and nifedipine.
  - Spironolactone.
  - Ciclosporin.

Evidence base

DIG Study (the effect of digoxin on mortality and morbidity in patients with heart failure)

Design: Double-blind RCT of digoxin versus placebo
Subjects: n = 6800; NYHA I–III; LVEF ≤ 45%; mean age = 63 years; 78% ♂
Follow-up: 37 months
Results: No significant difference in mortality (p = 0.80)
6% RRR in hospitalization (p = 0.01)
Reference: The effect of digoxin on mortality and morbidity in patients with heart failure. The Digitalis Investigation Group. *N Engl J Med* 1997; **336**: 525–33.

▶ Patients with AF were excluded from the DIG study.
Post-hoc analyses of DIG study suggest:
• Digoxin therapy is associated with an increased risk of all-cause mortality in women (23% relative risk increase, p = 0.014), but not men. Rathore SS, Wang Y, Krumholz HM. Sex-based differences in the effect of digoxin for the treatment of heart failure. *N Engl J Med* 2002; **347**: 1403–11.
• Higher serum digoxin concentrations (SDC) are associated with increased mortality in men. The authors suggest a SDC of 0.64–1nmol/L (0.5–0.8ng/mL). Rathore SS *et al.* Association of serum digoxin concentration and outcomes in patients with heart failure. *JAMA* 2003; **289**: 871–8.

Phosphodiesterase inhibitors

Phosphodiesterase inhibitors inhibit cAMP breakdown, with inotropic and vasodilatory effects. However, in large-scale placebo-controlled trials in patients with CHF, selective type III phosphodiesterase inhibitors (PDEI) were associated with an increase in mortality. Their use is, therefore, kept to short-term administration in decompensated patients in a critical care setting.

Properties
- Reduce after-load.
- Decrease filling pressures.
- Increase cardiac index.
- Increase the rate of contractility and relaxation.

Undesirable effects
- Increased mortality with long-term use.
- Pro-arrhythmic.

Pharmacology
- Enoximone
  - Variable elimination half-life (3–8 hours in HF patients).
  - 85% protein-bound.
  - Metabolized in the liver and excreted in the urine mainly as metabolites.
- Milrinone
  - Elimination half-life of 2–3 hours.
  - 70% protein-bound.
  - Elimination mainly in the urine (83% unchanged drug).

Administration
- Enoximone:
  - By intravenous infusion, initially 90µg/kg/minute over 10–30 minutes, followed by continuous infusion of 5–20µg/kg/minute.
  - Total dose over 24 hours should not usually exceed 24mg/kg.
- Milrinone:
  - By intravenous injection, 50µg/kg over 10 minutes followed by intravenous infusion at a rate of 375–750ng/kg/minute, if blood pressure satisfactory.
  - Maximum daily dose 1.13mg/kg.
  - Lower dose in renal impairment.

Evidence base

The PROMISE Study

Design: Double-blind RCT of oral milrinone versus placebo

Subjects: n = 1088; NYHA III–IV

Follow-up: 6.1 months

Results: 28% increase in mortality in patients treated with milrinone
(p = 0.038)

34% increase in cardiovascular mortality (p = 0.016)

53% increase in mortality in NYHA IV patients (p = 0.006)

Reference: Packer et al. Effect of oral milrinone on mortality in severe
chronic heart failure. The PROMISE Study Research Group.
N Engl J Med 1991; **325**: 1468–75.

OPTIME-CHF

Design: Double-blind RCT of IV milrinone versus placebo in patients
with an acute exacerbation of CHF

Subjects: n = 951; Mean age = 66 years; 93% NYHA III/IV; mean
LVEF = 23%

Follow-up: 60 days

Results: No difference in length of hospital stay, and in-hospital or
60-day mortality

More frequent hypotension (p < 0.001) and atrial arrhythmias
(p = 0.004) with milrinone

Reference: Cuffe MS et al. Short-term intravenous milrinone for acute
exacerbation of chronic heart failure: a randomized
controlled trial. JAMA 2002; **287**: 1541–7.

Calcium channel sensitizers

Levosimendan

Levosimendan is a calcium-sensitizing agent that promotes inotropy by stabilizing troponin C in a configuration which enhances the calcium sensitivity of cardiac myofilaments. Furthermore, levosimendan also leads to vasodilatation via the opening of ATP-dependent potassium channels. These two properties have led to the term 'inodilator'.

▶ Levosimendan is currently not licensed in the UK, but has been launched in the USA and parts of Europe.

Properties
- Inotropic.
- Vasodilatation.
- Reduces PCWP.
- Active metabolites may exert action for 5–7 days after treatment discontinued.

Undesirable effects
- Pro-arrhythmic (particularly atrial fibrillation).
- Headache.
- Hypotension.
- May increase long-term mortality.

Pharmacokinetics
Levosimendan is:
- 98% bound to plasma protein.
- Undergoes complete metabolism, with some active metabolites.
- Eliminination $t_{1/2}$-life is approximately 1 hour.

Administration (where licensed)
Given intravenously:
- Loading dose—12–24µg/kg over 10 minutes, followed by:
- Maintenance dose—IV infusion of 0.05–0.2µg/kg/minute, titrated to response.

Evidence base

LIDO study (levosimendan infusion versus dobutamine study)

Design: Double-blind RCT of levosimendan versus placebo

Subjects: n = 203; NYHA IV; LVEF ≤ 35%; mean age = 59 years; 87% ♂

Follow-up: 6 months

Results: 12% absolute (43% RRR) lower mortality with levosimendan compared with dobutamine at 6 months (p = 0.029)

13% (90% RRR) more patients had haemodynamic improvement at 24 hours with levosimendan compared with dobutamine (p = 0.022)

Reference: Follath F et al. Efficacy and safety of intravenous levosimendan compared with dobutamine in severe low-output heart failure (the LIDO study): a randomised double-blind trial. Lancet 2002; **360**: 196–202.

REVIVE-II (randomized multi-centre evaluation of intravenous levosimendan efficacy versus placebo in the short-term treatment of decompensated heart failure)

Design: Double-blind RCT of levosimendan versus placebo

Subjects: n = 600; HF admission; LVEF ≤ 35%; mean age = 63 years; 72% ♂

Follow-up: 6 months

Results: Trend to an increase in mortality at 90 days

Reduction in hospitalization by 2 days (p = 0.001)

More reports of hypotension and atrial fibrillation

Reference: AHA scientific sessions 2005.

SURVIVE

Design: Double-blind RCT of levosimendan versus dobutamine

Subjects: n = 1327; AHF with LVEF ≤ 30%; mean age = 59 years; 87% ♂

Follow-up: 180 days

Results: No significant difference in mortality at 180 days (p = 0.40)

Reference: Mebazaa A et al. Levosimendan vs dobutamine for patients with acute decompensated heart failure: the SURVIVE Randomized Trial. JAMA 2007; **297**: 1883–91.

PERSIST

Phase 2 study of oral form of levosimendan in approximately 300 patients with severe CHF failed to improve clinical outcomes; therefore, phase 3 study not proposed.

Vasodilators

Nesiritide

Nesiritide is recombinant human B-type natriuretic peptide, manufactured from *Escherichia coli*. It has the same 32-amino acid sequence as the endogenous peptide, which is produced by the ventricular myocardium. It is not licensed for use in the UK.

Mechanism of action

Endogenous BNP binds to the guanylate cyclase receptor of vascular smooth muscle and endothelial cells, leading to increased intracellular concentrations of cyclic GMP and smooth muscle cell relaxation. Thus, nesiritide causes dose-dependent reductions in pulmonary capillary wedge pressure (PCWP) and systemic arterial pressure by venous and arterial dilatation.

Clinical effects

- ↓ PCWP.
- ↓ After-load and pre-load.

Undesirable effects

- Hypotension.
- Possible renal dysfunction.

Pharmacokinetics

- Half-life ($t_{1/2}$) of approximately 18 minutes.
- Cleared from the circulation by:
  - Binding to cell surface clearance receptors with subsequent cellular internalization and lysosomal proteolysis.
  - Proteolytic cleavage of the peptide by endopeptidases, such as neutral endopeptidase.
  - Renal filtration.

Administration

- Intravenous infusion of 0.01–0.03µg/kg/minute.

Clinical trial evidence base
VMAC (vasodilation in the management of acute CHF)
Design: Double-blind RCT of nesiritide versus nitroglycerine versus
placebo

Subjects: n = 489; NYHA II–IV; mean age = 62 years; 69% ♂

Results: At 24 hours:

No significant difference in perceived dyspnoea

Greater reduction in PCWP with nesiritide (p = 0.04)

Reference: VMAC investigators. Intravenous nesiritide vs nitroglycerin
for treatment of decompensated congestive heart failure: a
randomized controlled trial. *JAMA* 2002; **287**: 1531–40.

▶ Nesiritide may significantly increase the risk of worsening renal
function and short-term mortality in patients with AHF (Sackner-
Bernstein JD *et al*. Risk of worsening renal function with nesiritide in
patients with acutely decompensated heart failure. *Circulation* 2005;
111: 1487–91 and Sackner-Bernstein JD *et al*. Short-term risk of death
after treatment with nesiritide for decompensated heart failure: a
pooled analysis of randomized controlled trials. *JAMA* 2005; **293**:
1900–5). For this reason, a large multi-centre study has been proposed
to clarify this, and is due to start recruiting in 2007.

Sodium nitroprusside

Sodium nitroprusside (SNP) causes peripheral vasodilation by a direct action on vascular smooth muscle. Prolonged administration may be associated with toxicity from its metabolites, thiocyanide and cyanide, and should be avoided especially in patients with severe renal or hepatic failure.

SNP should be uptitrated cautiously with invasive arterial monitoring. Likewise, SNP should be downtitrated slowly to avoid rebound hypertension. Controlled trials with SNP in AHF are lacking, and its administration in AMI has yielded equivocal results. In AHF caused by acute coronary syndromes, nitrates are favoured over SNP as SNP may cause 'coronary steal syndrome'.

Clinical effects
- Vasodilatation—reduction in both pre- and after-load.

Undesirable effects
- Hypotension.
- Headache.
- Nausea.

Pharmacokinetics
Sodium nitroprusside is rapidly metabolized and excreted entirely as metabolites, principally thiocyanate. The elimination half-life of thiocyanate is 2.7–7 days when renal function is normal, but is longer in patients with impaired renal function or hyponatraemia. Toxic symptoms begin to appear at plasma thiocyanate concentrations of 50–100µg/mL, and fatalities have been reported at concentrations of 200µg/mL.

Administration
- Intravenous infusion of 0.3–5µg/kg/minute uptitrating carefully.

Hydralazine

Hydralazine is principally an arteriolar dilator, although it has an uncertain mode of action. It has been shown to increase cardiac output with little effect on filling pressures. Hydralazine can also reduce the degree of mitral regurgitation. It is used in combination with isosorbide dinitrate (ISDN) in moderate to severe chronic heart failure in:

- Patients intolerant to ACE inhibitors or ARBs.
- African-Americans already established on ACE inhibitors or ARBs.

Clinical effects

- ↓ After-load.
- ↑ Cardiac output.

Undesirable effects

- Tachycardia.
- Fluid retention (renin release).
- Headache.
- Lupus syndrome (more likely to develop in slow acetylators).

Pharmacokinetics

- Rapidly absorbed from the gut (peak concentration 1–2 hours).
- Bioavailability: 26–55%.
- Peak plasma concentrations: 0.5–1.5 hours.
- Plasma protein binding: 90%.
- $t\frac{1}{2}$: 2–3 hours (but up to 16 hours in severe renal failure (CrCl<20 mL/minute, therefore reduce dose).
- Largely excreted as acetylated and hydroxylated metabolites, some of which are conjugated with glucuronic acid.

Administration

- Aim to uptitrate every 2 weeks if tolerated, paying particular caution in severe heart failure or in hypotensive patients:
- Starting dose: Hydralazine 25mg qds and isosorbide dinitrate 10mg qds
  Target dose: Hydralazine 75mg qds and isosorbide dinitrate 40mg qds.

Clinical trial evidence base

V-HeFT I (veterans administration cooperative study)

Design: Double-blind RCT of hydralazine/ISDN versus prazosin versus placebo

Subjects: n = 642; mean age = 58 years; 100% ♂; mean LVEF = 30%

Background therapy: diuretic and digoxin

Mean follow-up: 2.3 years

Results: 34% RRR in all-cause mortality for hydralazine/ISDN
(p = 0.028)

Reference: Cohn JN et al. Effect of vasodilator therapy on mortality in chronic congestive heart failure. Results of a veterans administration cooperative study. N Engl J Med 1986; **314**: 1547–52.

V-HeFT II

Design: Double-blind RCT of hydralazine and ISDN versus enalapril

Subjects: n = 804; mean age = 61 years; 100%♂; mean LVEF = 29%;
NYHA II/III

Background therapy: diuretic and digoxin

Mean follow-up: 2.5 years

Results: 28% RRR in all-cause mortality for enalapril (p = 0.016)

Reference: Cohn JN et al. A comparison of enalapril with hydralazine-isosorbide dinitrate in the treatment of chronic congestive heart failure. N Engl J Med 1991; **325**: 303–10.

A-HeFT I (African-American heart failure trial)

Design: Double-blind RCT of hydralazine/ISDN versus prazosin versus placebo

Subjects: n = 1050; mean age = 57 years; 60%♂; mean LVEF = 24%;
NYHA III/IV

Background therapy: 69% ACE-I; 74% β-blocker; 39% spironolactone

Mean follow-up: 2.3 years

Results: Terminated early

43% RRR in all-cause mortality (p = 0.01)

33% RRR in rate of first hospitalization (p = 0.001)

Improved quality of life

Reference: Taylor AL et al. Combination of isosorbide dinitrate and hydralazine in blacks with heart failure. N Engl J Med 2004; **351**: 2049–57.

Nitrates

Nitrates relieve pulmonary congestion in acute heart failure by increasing vasodilatory cyclic GMP in vascular smooth muscle. At low doses, nitrates principally induce venodilation, but as the dose increases they cause arterial dilation.

Clinical effects

- ↓ Pre-load.
- ↓ After-load.
- ↓ Myocardial oxygen demand.

Undesirable effects

- Headache.
- Hypotension.

Pharmacokinetics

Exposure to nitrates result in the rapid development of tolerance (particularly when given IV in high doses), limiting their effectiveness to 16–24 hours.

- Glyceryl trinitrate.
  - Large volume of distribution.
  - Rapidly metabolized to dinitrates and mononitrates.
  - $t_{1/2}$: 1–4 minutes.
  - 30–60% plasma protein bound.
  - The principal metabolite is glyceryl mononitrate, which is inactive.
- Isosorbide dinitrate (ISDN).
  - Bioavailability: 80% (oral).
  - $t_{1/2}$: 2 hours (oral).
  - $t_{1/2}$: 0.7 hours (IV).
  - Metabolized to active metabolites (isosorbide mononitrate).

Administration

Nitrates should be administered with careful BP monitoring. The dose should be reduced if systolic blood pressure falls <90mmHg, and discontinued permanently if blood pressure drops further.

- s/l 2 puffs (400µg) of glyceryl trinitrate every 5 minutes.
- buccal 1–5mg of isosorbide dinitrate.
- IV GTN 20–200µg/minute or isosorbide dinitrate 1–10mg/hour.

Clinical trial evidence base

Design: RCT of high-dose ISDN and low-dose furosemide versus high-dose furosemide and low-dose ISDN in AHF

Subjects: n = 104; mean age = 74 years; 52% ♂; mean LVEF = 42%

Background therapy: 87% ACE-I; 50% β-blocker

Results: Less requirement for mechanical ventilation (p = 0.0041) and fewer MI (p = 0.047) in high-dose ISDN group

Reference: Cotter G *et al.* Randomised trial of high-dose isosorbide dinitrate plus low-dose furosemide versus high-dose furosemide plus low-dose isosorbide dinitrate in severe pulmonary oedema. *Lancet* 1998; **351**: 389–93.

Section VI

How to set up and run a heart failure service

Heart failure services

Introduction

The management of HF due to systolic dysfunction is underpinned by one of the strongest evidence bases in medicine. Following large randomized drug treatment trials of ACE inhibitors and β-adrenoreceptor antagonists published in the late 1980s and early 1990s, numerous guidelines have been written (ESC, ACC/AHA, NHFA/CSANZ, SIGN, and NICE). Despite this, registry data show a low uptake of these therapies in the community, and both morbidity and mortality remain high. This has led to a paradigm shift away from individual drug therapies, to the systems of care in which treatments are delivered, that is, within organized multi-professional heart failure services.

Complexity of HF

The need for multi-professional HF services arises from the increasing complexity of diagnosing and managing HF. Patients are asked to make lifestyle changes, take multiple drugs, and are increasingly exposed to device therapy. In addition, the average age of a HF patient at diagnosis is 76 years—that is, it is predominantly a 'cardiogeriatric syndrome'. Patients affected have frequent and multiple co-morbidities, and the therapies themselves have numerous side-effects.

In the midst of all this, the HF patient has to make multiple visits to hospital clinics, often seeing numerous doctors. This can sow the seeds for enormous confusion likely to result in patchy adherence to therapy.

Evidence for heart failure services

Several RCTs of multi-professional versus usual care have now been carried out. Seminal ones include:
- Rich *et al.* 1995 (Fig. 38.1)
  - Nurse directed multi-professional HF intervention versus usual care in HF patients aged >70 years at high risk of re-admission.
  - The interventional arm included education, dietary advice, cardiology review, home visits, and telephone contact.
  - 44% reduction in all-cause re-admissions at 90 days (p = 0.035).
- Stewart *et al.* 1999 (Fig. 38.2)
  - Randomized patients to usual care versus home visit from nurse for education about medication after an admission for HF.
  - Significant reduction in event-free survival at 1 year (p = 0.037).
- Blue *et al.* 2001 (Fig. 38.3)
  - 165 admissions with HF, randomized to nurse intervention/usual care.
  - ↓ All-cause admissions (86 versus 114, p = 0.018).
  - ↓ HF admissions (19 versus 45, p < 0.001).
  - Fewer days in hospital for HF (3.43 versus 7.46, p = 0.0051).

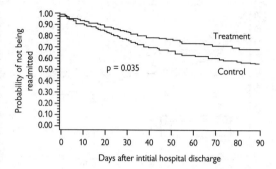

Fig. 38.1 Kaplan–Kaplan curve for the probability of not being re-admitted to the hospital during the 90-day period of follow-up. Reproduced from Rich M *et al.* A multidisciplinary intervention to prevent the readmission of elderly patients with congestive heart failure. *N Engl J Med* 1995; **333**: 1190–5 with permission from Massacheussets Medical Society.

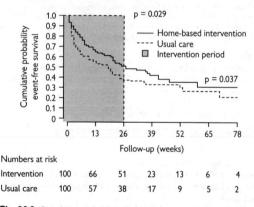

Fig. 38.2 Cumulative probability of event-free survival during follow-up. Reproduced from Stewart S *et al.* Effects of a multidisciplinary, home-based intervention on unplanned readmissions and survival among patients with chronic congestive heart failure: a randomised controlled study. *Lancet* 1999; **354**: 1077–83 with permission from Elsevier.

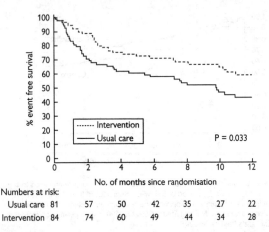

Numbers at risk:

Usual care	81	57	50	42	35	27	22
Intervention	84	74	60	49	44	34	28

Fig. 38.3 Time to first event (death from any cause or hospital admission or heart failure) in usual care and nurse intervention groups. Reproduced from Blue LM et al. Randomised controlled trial of specialist nurse intervention in heart failure. *BMJ* 2001; **323**: 715 with permission from *BMJ* Publishing Group Ltd.

Other evidence

Numerous other trials of multidisciplinary strategies have been reported, but they are heterogeneous in terms of the models of care they have employed. Models have included:
- Multi-professional HF clinics.
- Multi-disciplinary follow-up without HF clinics.
- Telephone contact.
- Primary care follow-up.
- Enhanced patient self-care.

A systematic review of 29 trials showed:
- Specialized multidisciplinary team (clinic or non-clinic setting): reduced mortality (↓ 25%), and both HF (↓ 26%) and all-cause (↓ 19%) hospitalizations.
- Enhanced patient self-care: reduced HF (↓ 34%) and all-cause hospitalizations (↓ 27%).
- Telephone contact, with referral to GP if further help advised, reduced HF hospitalizations (↓ 25%).
- Higher prescribing/dosing of disease-modifying therapy.
- Improved drug compliance.
- Most strategies were cost-saving.

Guidelines

Most society guidelines (ACC/AHA/NHFA/CSANZ/NICE/SIGN) now state that HF care should be delivered in a multi-professional manner.

Essential components

Most HF services have unique features specific to their geographical location, disease prevalence, local resources, and barriers to optimal care. Many are evolving into HF networks to provide comprehensive care for a community. Essential components seem to include:

- Specially trained HF nurses have a role in educating the patient about HF and its precipitating factors, dietary advice, and the need for compliance with therapy.
- Access to clinicians trained in HF.

Key references

Hunt SA et al. ACC/AHA 2005 Guideline update for the diagnosis and management of chronic heart failure in the adult. *J Am Coll Cardiol* 2005; **46**(6): e1–82.

Krum H et al. Guidelines for the prevention, detection and management of people with chronic heart failure in Australia 2006. *Med J Aust* 2006; **185**: 549–56.

McAlister FA et al. Multidisciplinary strategies for the management of heart failure patients at high risk for admission: a systematic review of randomized trials. *J Am Coll Cardiol* 2004; **44**: 810–19.

NICE Guideline for Heart Failure. www.nice.org.uk/guidance/CG5

Swedberg K et al. Guidelines for the diagnosis and treatment of chronic heart failure: executive summary (update 2005): The Task Force for the Diagnosis and Treatment of Chronic Heart Failure of the European Society of Cardiology. *Eur Heart J* 2005; **26**: 1115–40.

Towards HF networks

A multi-professional HF service must:
- Have local guidelines to be used across all levels of care.
- Be able to manage HF in both primary and secondary care to ensure consistency of approach.
- Include medical therapy guidelines that can be used to allow nurse prescribing and optimization of therapy.
- These should be based around the existing practice guidelines for the management of CHF (e.g. ESC/AHA/NHFA/CSANZ/SIGN/ NICE).

Ideally, a HF service should be centred on a HF clinic. The HF clinic should:
- Be multidisciplinary: involving cardiologists, GPs, care of the elderly physicians, specialist nurses, and pharmacists, as appropriate.
- Provide a supportive milieu for health care professionals (HCPs).
- Provide places for supervision and training.
- Facilitate better time management for nurses with patients who are able to attend compared with more time-consuming home visits.
- Allow rapid access to heart failure expertise for primary and secondary care physicians, other specialist HCPs, and patients.

The aims of such a service are to:
- Provide an accurate diagnosis.
- Instigate appropriate investigation.
- Roll out a management plan.

A heart failure service should be available to the HF patient wherever they enter their health care journey, whether that is in primary care, as a HF admission to an internal medicine ward, or the CCU, or as a referral to secondary or tertiary care.

The management for most patients will be rolled out in primary care, aided by HF nurses, and cardiology liaison from secondary/tertiary care. Some patients need to attend HF clinics for more intensive management, and others require access to advanced HF care for the consideration of device therapy and rarer and more rationed therapies, such as cardiac transplantation and LV assist devices. Selected patients will require palliative care services. The aim of a HF service is to improve the outcomes for all HF patients, regardless of their entry point to health care (see Fig. 38.4).

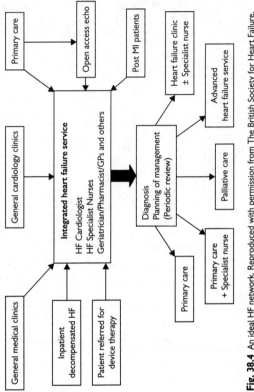

Fig. 38.4 An ideal HF network. Reproduced with permission from The British Society for Heart Failure.

Section VII

End of life issues

Palliative care

The need for palliative care in HF

Palliative care, or 'End-of-Life Therapies' for HF, really refers to a shift in the focus of care from management primarily aimed at prolonging life to that concerned chiefly with the relief of symptoms.

Mortality and morbidity of advanced HF

According to the HF treatment trials, the annual mortality rate of HF due to systolic dysfunction, when we look at the incremental effects of disease-modifying therapy, is now around 7% per annum.

Despite this, HF remains a fatal disease for most patients—as they are not representative of those enrolled in the landmark trials. These real-world HF patients are much older (mean age at diagnosis of 76 years) and have frequent co-morbidities. Their mortality rates are greater than those of the most common cancers—diseases for which there is well-established palliative care. Indeed, the mortality rates from a recent trial in advanced HF (REMATCH) are striking:

- 75% 1-year mortality for those randomized to medical therapy.
- Greater in those intolerant of ACEI and/or BB.

The median survival for inotrope-dependent patients is 3.2 months.
The mortality or re-hospitalization rates in advanced HF are 81% at 1 year.

Symptoms are frequent and include

- Lack of energy.
- Breathlessness (60%).
- Weakness or fatigue.
- Pain—78% (comparable to lung/colon cancer).
- Insomnia.
- Depression.

Patient's and carer's view

Boyd and co-workers studied how patients and their carers viewed health and social care in the last year of life in NHYA IV HF. They conducted serial interviews with 20 patients, 27 carers, and 30 health care professionals. They found that quality of life was severely reduced by physical and psychological morbidity. In addition, psychosocial care, patient and carer education, and coordination of care between primary and secondary care were poor. A palliative care approach was rare.

Key references

Boyd K et al. Living with advanced heart failure: a prospective, community based study of patients and their carers. *Eur J Heart Fail* 2004; **6**: 585–91.

Croft JB et al. Heart failure survival among older adults in the United States: a poor prognosis for an emerging epidemic in the Medicare population. *Arch Intern Med* 1999; **159**: 505–10.

Hershberger RE et al. Care processes and clinical outcomes of continuous outpatient support with inotropes (COSI) in patients with refractory endstage heart failure. *J Card Fail* 2003; **9**: 180–7.

Rose EA et al. Long-term mechanical left ventricular assistance for end-stage heart failure. *N Engl J Med* 2001; **345**: 1435–43.

Timing

Disease progression in heart failure

Timing of palliative care in HF is difficult. The disease trajectory is fundamentally different to cancers, where there is often a fairly predictable and inexorable decline towards death once response to treatment fails. In HF, half of all the patients die suddenly, although this proportion is smaller in those with advanced heart failure where most succumb to progressive pump failure (see Fig. 39.1).

Despite a plethora of prognostic markers in HF, none provide much help on their own for deciding when palliative care should begin, although they can help provide confirmatory evidence of advanced disease.

For whom?

Palliative care should be considered for those with:
- Severe functional limitation
- End organ hypoperfusion, despite optimized medical therapy
- Significant disease progression in the previous 6 months:
  - Multiple hospital admissions
  - Loss of ability to perform activities of daily living
  - No remediable/exacerbating factors
  - Ineligible for transplantation/assist device.

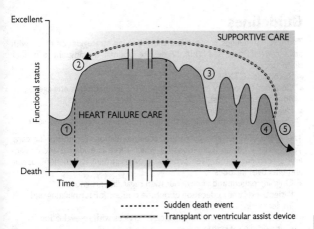

Fig. 39.1 The disease trajectory in HF. Schematic course of stage C and D heart failure. The stages refer to the ACC/AHA Classification Stages of HF—Stage C: patients with left ventricular dysfunction and with current or prior symptoms; Stage D: end stage. Sudden death may occur at any point along the course of illness. (1) Initial symptoms of heart failure (HF) develop, and HF treatment is initiated. (2) Plateaus of variable length may be reached with initial medical management, or after mechanical support, or heart transplant. (3) Functional status declines with variable slope, with intermittent exacerbations of HF that respond to rescue efforts. (4) Stage D HF, with refractory symptoms and limited function. (5) End-of-life. Reproduced from Goodlin S *et al.* Consensus statement: Palliative and supportive care in advanced heart failure. *J Card Fail* 2004; **10**: 200–9 with permission from Heart Failure Society of America.

Guidelines

The ESC Guidelines recommend the following strategies for those with advanced HF, that is, NYHA IV despite optimal therapy and a proper diagnosis.

- Reconsider CTX-unlikely for the vast majority.
- Consider temporary inotropic support (IV sympathomimetic agents, dopaminergic agonist, and/or phoshodiesterase inhibitors).
- Palliative treatment in terminal patients should always be considered, and may include the use of opiates for symptoms relief.

The AHA/ACC has also published recommendations for end-of-life care. Their 'class I' advice (conditions for which there is evidence and/or general agreement that a given procedure or treatment is beneficial, useful, and effective) includes

- Ongoing patient and family education regarding prognosis.
- Patient and family education about the options for formulating and implementing advance directives.
- A role for palliative and hospice care services with re-evaluation for changing clinical status.
- Discussion regarding the option of inactivating ICDs.
- Ensuring continuity of medical care between inpatient and outpatient areas.
- Components of hospice care that are appropriate to the relief of suffering, including opiates, are recommended, and they do not exclude the options for use of inotropes and IV diuretics for symptom palliation.

Managing end-stage HF

Conventional HF therapy

This is difficult—especially in considering which drugs to stop as many disease-modifying drugs for HF also reduce symptoms. These include

- Digoxin.
- Diuretics.
- ACE inhibitors.
- Angiotensin receptor antagonists.
- β-adrenoreceptor antagonists.
- Spironolactone.

In general, these should be continued but may require reduction or cessation if they are causing symptomatic hypotension, tiredness, or renal dysfunction.

Devices

- CRT improves HF symptoms in NYHA III/IV subjects.
- ICDs can alter the mode of death from sudden to progressive pump failure. Consideration should be given to switching the defibrillation function off after discussion with the patient and their family.

Specific palliative therapies—breathlessness

Morphine: Evidence from a small ($n = 10$) RCT, with a double-blinded crossover design in NYHA III/IV HF subjects, using 5mg oral morphine 4-hourly, demonstrated a significant reduction in breathlessness without any adverse effect in terms of sedation. 2.5mg morphine was used if the serum creatinine was >200μmol/L. The treatment was combined with an anti-emetic haloperidol 1.5mg at night and lactulose if necessary (see Fig. 39.2).

Oxygen: A small study showed that oxygen therapy improved dyspnoea, but not effort or functional capacity.

Oral inotropes

- Can improve dyspnoea and exercise tolerance, but decrease survival (there have been mixed results for enoximone and pimonendan).
- Low-dose oral enoximone and β-blockade, increased functional capacity.
- The ESSENTIAL study, RCT of oral enoximone versus placebo in NYHA III/IV HF, demonstrated no increase in mortality with enoximone and an increase in exercise duration and trend to improved symptoms.

IV inotropes

- Are used infrequently in the community in Europe, there is more experience in the USA.
- They are usually used in hospitalized HF patients with a low cardiac output.
- They can provide symptomatic relief.
- In those who are inotrope dependent, that is, cannot be weaned, home IV support is an option in some areas.

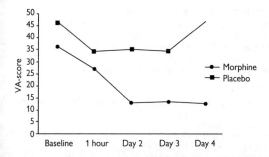

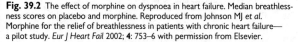

Fig. 39.2 The effect of morphine on dyspnoea in heart failure. Median breathlessness scores on placebo and morphine. Reproduced from Johnson MJ *et al.* Morphine for the relief of breathlessness in patients with chronic heart failure—a pilot study. *Eur J Heart Fail* 2002; **4**: 753–6 with permission from Elsevier.

Key references

ESSENTIAL Investigators ESC 2005.

Kubo SH. Effects of pimobendan on exercise tolerance and quality of life in patients with heart failure. *Cardiology* 1997; **88**: 21–7.

Lowes BD *et al.* Low-dose enoximone improves exercise capacity in chronic heart failure. Enoximone Study Group. *J Am Coll Cardiol* 2000; **36**: 501–8.

Russell SD *et al.* Lack of effect of increased inspired oxygen concentrations on maximal exercise capacity or ventilation in stable heart failure. *Am J Cardiol* 1999; **84**: 1412–16.

Utretsky BF *et al.* Multicenter trial of oral enoximone in patients with moderate to moderately severe congestive heart failure. Lack of benefit compared with placebo. Enoximone Multicenter Trial Group. *Circulation* 1990; **82**:774–80.

Specific palliative therapies—tiredness
- Sleep-disordered breathing occurs in 50% of advanced HF.
- Some studies show that CPAP can improve LV function and neurohormonal profile in central sleep apnoea. This should be assessed and treated if necessary.
- The role of psychostimulants remains to be determined.

Delivery of care

Interdisciplinary supportive care should be delivered. The key features are:
- Communication is essential.
- End-of-life planning is required.
- Concurrent with 'multi-professional HF' care.
- Should focus on patients and families.

The SUPPORT study demonstrated that 50% of seriously ill hospitalized patients, who survived 10 days, preferred care focused on comfort. Most patients prefer quality of life rather than longevity.

The palliative care given should relieve symptoms and provide holistic interdisciplinary support for patients and family. It can occur in several settings:
- Home based.
- Integrated HF care.
- Hospice based.

How to deliver care

How best to deliver end-of-life care causes anxiety and confusion for health care professionals. Should all end-stage HF patients be referred to a palliative care physician? This is clearly impractical, despite the fact that non-cancer palliative care is increasing. They would be unable to cope with the numbers. However, access to a palliative care consultative service is essential for those patients who require it.

The St George's experience of integrated HF care demonstrates a good model of care delivery. They studied 121 consecutive deaths between 1999 and 2002 in their hospital, with the following outcome:
- They developed a model of integrated, consultative, palliative care within a comprehensive HF management programme.
- They empowered HF nurse specialists, GPs, cardiologists, and internists to deliver palliative care.
- Ultimately, only 8.3% needed formal palliative care, 2.5% needed community palliative care services, and 4.1% hospice care (Figs 39.3 and 39.4).

Palliative care consultation arrangements should be integrated into the existing multidisciplinary HF management programmes, so that this important end-of-life care can be delivered to those who need it.

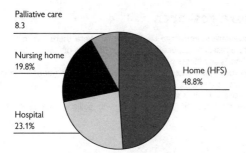

Fig. 39.3 The St George's integrated palliative care service—place of death of patients in collaborative heart failure program. HFS indicates Heart Failure Service (a community-based heart failure disease management program). Reproduced from Davidson et al. Integrated, collaborative palliative care in heart failure: the St. George Heart Failure Service experience 1999–2002. *J Cardiovasc Nurs* 2004; **19**: 68–75 with permission from Lippincott, Williams and Wilkins. SUPPORT Investigators JAMA 1995; **274**: 1591

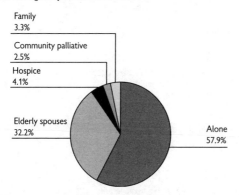

Fig. 39.4 The St George's integrated palliative care service—level of support for patients in a home based collaborative care program. Reproduced from Davidson et al. Integrated, collaborative palliative care in heart failure: the St. George Heart Failure Service experience 1999–2002. *J Cardiovasc Nurs* 2004; **19**: 68–75 with permission from Lippincott, Williams and Wilkins.

Key references

A controlled trial to improve care for seriously ill hospitalized patients. The study to understand prognoses and preferences for outcomes and risks of treatments (SUPPORT). The SUPPORT Principal Investigators. *JAMA* 1995; **274**: 1591–8.

Kohnlein T et al. Central sleep apnoea syndrome in patients with chronic heart disease: a critical review of the current literature. *Thorax* 2002; **57**: 547–54.

Lenique F et al. Ventilatory and hemodynamic effects of continuous positive airway pressure in left heart failure. *Am J Respir Crit Care Med* 1997; **155**: 500–5.

Naughton MT et al. Effects of nasal CPAP on sympathetic activity in patients with heart failure and central sleep apnea. *Am J Respir Crit Care Med* 1995; **152**: 473–9.

Future research

Palliative care in end-stage HF is an area where there has to be a focus on future research, especially within the domains of:

- Prognosis and illness trajectory.
- Symptom treatments, for example, opioids, interventions for fatigue, and antidepressants.
- Patient and family support.
- Models of integration of HF services with palliative care services.

Index